John McDougall, the doctor who fought for you

by Peter Rogers MD, copyright © August 2024.

Subtitle: The greatest doctor who ever lived

Cover painting is "God Speed!" by Edmund Leighton, 1900, public domain.

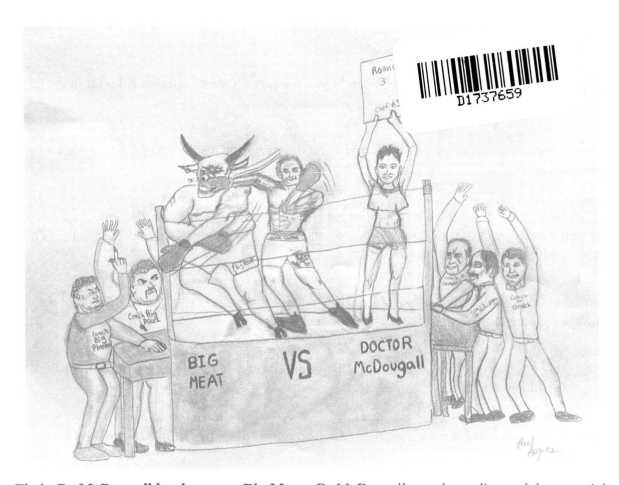

Fig i: Dr McDougall lands one on Big Meat. Dr McDougall was the undisputed, heavyweight champion of the nutrition and health world for over 30 years. Drawing made by the author's friend, and given to author for his educational videos & books.

"People ask, "Can I ever be healthy again? I say, STARCH is the SOLUTION for how to become HEALTHY!... **All large, healthy populations eat a starch based diet.** There are no exceptions… Humans are starchivores…

Starch has unlocked the door to health for thousands of my patients… We humans are built to thrive on starch.

The more starch we consume, the healthier we become. I recommend that people get

about 90% of their calories from starch. You don't need to weigh it. Just eyeballing the amounts is fine.

Starches include rice, corn, potatoes, sweet potatoes, beans, peas, barley, millet, oats, quinoa, rye, sorghum, wheat, squash. If a person only ate white rice, they could get beri beri, but that's easy to prevent with just a little bit of fruits and vegetables.

If you take just one message from this book, it should be: **EAT MORE STARCH**...

I'm the luckiest doctor in the world, because my patients get well.

The fat you eat is the fat you wear... the higher the percentage of calories from fat in the diet; the fatter the population...

Fat is the major toxin in the Western diet... fat paralyzes the insulin receptor, and causes diabetes...

It's important for patients to realize that fat causes diabetes. How can a patient get better if they don't know that? If they don't know that, then they don't know what they should do. The key to resolving acne is to minimize dietary fat...

Fat causes red blood cells to stick together, which is called blood sludge; blood sludge is the main cause of hypertension... **High fat meal decreases PaO2 by 20%**

Blood sludge lowers oxygen delivery to the tissues... oils are even worse than saturated fat for causing blood sludge...

Best way to prevent or even reverse atherosclerosis is to **reduce the amount fat in the diet**...

All forms of dietary fat increase the risk of obesity, diabetes, and hypertension...

High fat diets increase the risk of leaky gut, and autoimmune disease...

A hot dog is a ground up animal. It contains thyroid tissue. This can lead to thyroid autoimmune disease...

There's plenty of omega 3's in low fat, plant foods... my concern about omega 3 supplements is that they suppress the immune system... there's considerable evidence that fish fat (omega 3 fat) will increase a person's risk of cancer, and also will increase the risk of metastasis... fish fat is known to paralyze the action of insulin (Mcdougall newsletter Feb 2003)

it's impossible for a diet to be too low in protein…

it's impossible for a diet to be too low in calcium…

I get asked, "Why are people so sick?" I tell them, **"It's the food!"**… Good health information gives people the opportunity to have a better life… The most important thing in medicine is the food. In order to get the cure, you must stop the cause!

The paleo, keto, low carb, high fat promoters have money on their side, but We [the low fat, starch based vegans] have the truth on our side… The truth don't change… .. People love to hear "good" news about their bad habits [so they feel free to continue eating them]…

This keto diet stuff reminds me of what PT barnum said, "There's a sucker born every minite.

The treadmill stress test is a conveyor belt to the cardiac cath lab, and the operating room… the "widow maker" coronary artery lesion is a "sales pitch." **Coronary artery stents do not extend life!** Not at all! I have a tattoo on my chest that says, "Do not cath!"

With asymptomatic patients, there is ZERO% benefit of screening colonoscopy [when the complications are subtracted from the benefits]…

Mastectomy doesn't add one day to your life over lumpectomy for breast cancer… **Starch is better than fruits for satisfying hunger.** There's no such thing as a fruitarian population… There's no large population that subsists primarily on fruits… fruits tend to be seasonal, and they don't store as well as starches… starches are better able to satisfy hunger than are fruits.

70% of nutrition and health literature is funded by industry. You can't trust it anymore…

When change your diet to low fat vegan, be prepared for a precipitous drop in blood pressure; & most type 2 diabetics will be able to come off their diabetes medications. My low fat diet for treatment of hypertension, does not allow high fat foods like oils, nuts, seeds, avocados.

Sick people take medications. Healthy people do not take medications. Sick people have surgical scars on their abdomen & chest. Sick people have regular doctor visits. You want to get out of the medical business. The only way to get out of the medical business is to stop being sick. The only way to stop being sick is to regain your health; to fix the problem. The problem is the food.

The McDougall diet is starch >> fruits and veggies, with no animal foods, and no oils. When you remove the animal foods and oils, you remove most of the fat. For patients trying to lose weight they should also avoid high fat plant foods like avocados, coconuts, nuts, seeds, and soy.

Starch helps people lose weight in three ways: 1. It's low in fat. 2. It has low caloric density. 3. It's the best food to satisfy hunger… Dietary fat does NOT satisfy hunger well at all.

With aging, a person does not have to develop obesity, hypertension, diabetes, and coronary artery disease. With the McDougall diet, people don't get those diseases...

Cooked foods are good. The so called benefits of raw foods, and that stuff about enzymes was exaggerated. Humans have eaten cooked starches for a very long time.

The human body is always trying to heal. Just give it the food it needs, starch. Get your sleep. Get some sunshine. Make yourself happy by helping other people…

The gladiators were barley men. Sweet potatos are probably the healthiest food…

Old people don't need more protein. Exercise is good for them.

The Atkins diet is the make yourself sick diet… the Kempner diet is the diet for the nearly dead… **the McDougall diet is for the living**…

Type 2 diabetes is 100% curable…Why manage type 2 diabetes with pills, when you can CURE IT with diet?" - John McDougall MD.

"The best way to categorize diets is by the amount of fat… there's no such thing as a diet that's too low in fat... I have reviewed the literature on dietary fat… fat causes lipotoxicity... **fat is bad**… almost all Americans are diabetic after dinner, because they eat a high fat diet…" - Nathan Pritikin, nutrition genius.

"The most common cause of disease is ignorance… It only took me two hours to become a vegan; two hours of talking to Dr McDougall" – Ruth Heidrich Phd, 40+ year survivor of metastatic breast cancer.

"Fat causes red blood cells to stick together, and a diet like this increases the risk of multiple sclerosis… the most important thing for preventing MS is to reduce the intake of saturated fat" – Roy Swank MD, neurologist with best results for treating MS.

"Eating a low protein diet lowers workload of kidneys" – Walter Kempner MD, rice diet.

"The only way we are going to restore our health is to go back to eating the plant based high fiber diets of our ancestors… People who eat high fiber diets have larger, softer stools. If the people have little stools, they need big hospitals." - Dennis Burkitt MD, pioneer of abdominal pressure syndrome.

Table of contents

Foreword   7
1. Introduction
2. Who is John McDougall?   8
3. Who is the greatest doctor ever?   45
4. Dr McDougall's medical achievements   53
5. Mentors – Burkitt, Kempner, Swank, Pritikin   68
6. The Starch Solution book   98
7. The Gastrointestinal tuneup book   105
8. Obesity and fat   112
9. Hypertension   128
10. Diabetes   134
11. Cancer   141
12. Autoimmune diseases & arthritis   151
13. Heart disease   162
14. Dementia   172
15. Kidneys & Osteoporosis   177
16. McDougall diet   187
17. McDougall FAQ's   189
18. The Potato   199
19. Dr McDougall quotes   203
20. References   215
21. About author   219
22. Index   224

Warning:

The low fat, 100% vegan, whole food, starch based diet with no oils has a powerful effect on health. If you are taking medicines for diabetes or hypertension, and possibly for other conditions, **YOU WILL MOST LIKELY NEED TO LOWER YOUR MEDICATION DOSAGES!** So, talk to your health care provider to help you adjust your medication dosages.

Dedication

To John and Mary McDougall,

Your unwavering dedication to truth in nutrition and health has illuminated the path for countless individuals, including myself. John, your tireless efforts to educate and empower patients have inspired generations of health conscious individuals and medical professionals alike. Mary, you steadfast support and culinary wisdom have made the journey to health, not just possible, but delicious.

This book is dedicated to you both, in gratitude for the lives you've changed, the truths you've championed, and the legacy of health you've created. Your work continues to ripple through time, touching lives and transforming health. May this compilation serve as a testament to your enduring impact on human health and happiness.

With deepest respect and appreciation,

Peter Rogers MD

	Sat fat	Oil	Sodium	Tob	Fruits & vegetables	Dm	Htn	MI	Stroke	Impotence	Cancer
American	High	mod	Moderate 6 g/d	Low	Low	Mod to high	Mod to High	High	Moderate	High	High
E. Asian, Japan, Korea, China	Low	Low	High > 12 g/d	High	Moderate	Low	High	Low	High		Moderate
S. Asian, India	Low to mod (dairy)	High	High	Low	Low	High	High	High	mod	High	
Low fat, low sodium, vegan	Low	ZERO	Low	ZERO	High	ZERO	ZERO	ZERO	Very low	Very low	Very low

Fig ii: Low fat, starch based vegans, with no oil, are the healthiest people, by far.

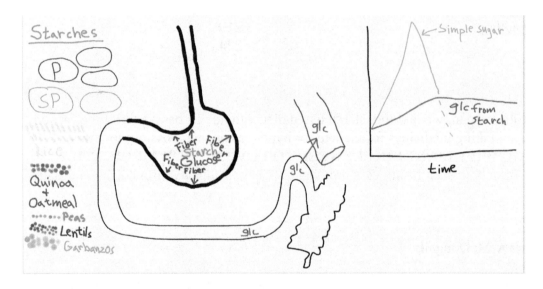

Fig iii: **Starch is the best food** to keep you healthy. **Starch is a polymer of glucose wrapped in fiber.** Starch is low caloric density, so it stretches the stomach (providing early satisfaction of hunger). The small bowel enzymes need time to gradually separate the fiber from the glucose. This leads to a slow & steady absorption of glucose from the gut to the blood. This keeps your blood glucose in the normal range for a prolonged amount of time. This **satisfies hunger with the fewest number of calories.** This optimizes body weight and health. **This is THE most important thing to know about health & nutrition.** "All long standing, healthy populations eat a starch based diet. There are no exceptions." – John McDougall MD.

Foreword

In the realm of nutrition and health, few voices have been as consistent, passionate, and influential as that of John McDougall MD. For decades, Dr McDougall has been a beacon of wisdom in a sea of conflicting health information, advocating for a simple yet revolutionary approach to diet and wellness. His message, grounded in scientific evidence and years of clinical experience, has transformed countless lives, including my own and those of my family.

Dr Peter Rogers has undertaken he monumental task of distilling Dr McDougall's life's work into this comprehensive volume. As a fellow physician with impressive credentials, Dr Rogers brings a keen analytical eye and deep understanding to McDougall's teachings. This book serves as both a tribute to Dr McDougall, and an invaluable resource for anyone seeking to understand and apply his principles.

What sets this book apart is its thoroughness. Dr Rogers has meticulously combed through McDougall's extensive body of work – from his ground breaking books, and newsletters, to his engaging video lectures, and the wealth of information at DrMcDougall.com. The result is a carefully curated collection of McDougall's most best insights, organized in a way that makes them accessible, and applicable.

Readers will find clear explanations of the **"Starch Solution,"** and why it forms the cornerstone of McDougall's dietary recommendations. The book examines McDougall's approach to **treating and reversing chronic diseases like heart disease, diabetes, and autoimmune conditions** through diet. It also captures Dr McDougall's sharp critiques of the medical establishment and the food industry.

One of the most valuable aspects of this book is how it preserves Dr McDougall's voice – his directness, his humor, and his unwavering commitment to empowering patients. Through carefully selected quotes and anecdotes, Dr Rogers brings McDougall's personality to life, allowing new readers to experience the charisma that has inspired so many.

Whether you're a longtime follower of Dr McDougall or new to his approach, this book offers something of value. For the initiated, it serves as a **comprehensive reference guide,** bringing together key concepts from across McDougall's career. For newcomers, it provides an excellent introduction to McDougall's philosophy, and practical advice.

In compiling this work, Dr Rogers has done a great service, not just to Dr McDougall's legacy, but to anyone seeking a clearer path to health. This book stands as a testament to the power of McDougall's message, and its enduring relevance in our modern world.

As you explore these pages, I hope you'll find, as I have, a wealth of knowledge that can transform your understanding of health and empower you to take control of your well being. Dr McDougall's life's work, so thoroughly presented here, has the potential to change – and save – countless lives. It is my pleasure to introduce you to this compendium of one of the great medical minds of our time.

Jeff Nelson
VegSource.com

Chapter 1. **Introduction**

The best place to go to learn about Dr McDougall's work, and telehealth center is his website, **"Dr McDougall dot com."**

You will see:

1. You can sign up for his telehealth or in person clinic which is run by his protege Dr Anthony Lim.
2. The legacy book of Nathan Pritikin, available free.
3. You will see the legacy book of Dr Walter Kempner, available free.
4. Numerous testimonials of patients cured by the McDougall diet, called Star McDougallers, including yours truly.
5. Dr McDougall's monthly nutrition newsletter, from 1986-2017, which is the best nutrition newsletter in the world.
6. The free version of his color picture book "Food Poisoning"
7. Numerous videos & written articles about common, and uncommon diseases.
8. Educational courses

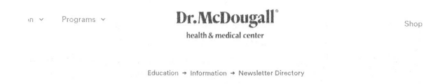

Dr.McDougall
health & medical center

Shop

Education → Information → Newsletter Directory

Newsletter Archives (2002-2017)

Search Legacy Content

Search archives for...

Search

Note: This opens up a Google Search for this website, and includes content from both our main site and our newsletters dating back to 1986.

2017	Jan, Feb, Mar	Apr, May, Jun	Jul, Aug, Sep	
2016	Jan, Feb, Mar	Apr, May, Jun	Jul, Aug, Sep	Oct, Nov, Dec
2015	Jan, Feb, Mar	Apr, May, Jun	Jul, Aug, Sep	Oct, Nov, Dec
2014	Jan, Feb, Mar	Apr, May, Jun	Jul, Aug, Sep	Oct, Nov, Dec
2013	Jan, Feb, Mar	Apr, May, Jun	Jul, Aug, Sep	Oct, Nov, Dec

Fig 1-1. Dr McDougall's newsletter archive at Dr McDougall dot com.

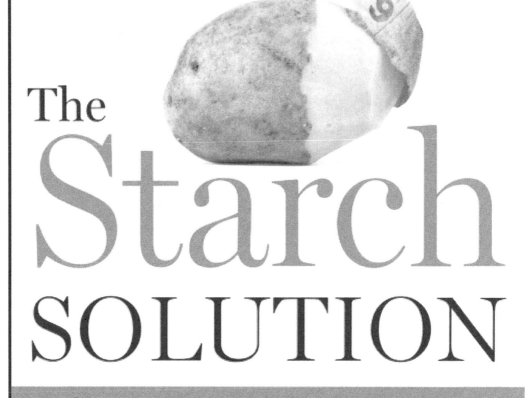

EAT THE FOODS YOU LOVE,
REGAIN YOUR HEALTH, AND
LOSE THE WEIGHT FOR GOOD!

The
Starch
SOLUTION

JOHN A. McDOUGALL, MD
AND MARY McDOUGALL

Fig 1-2: The Starch Solution by John McDougall MD & Mary McDougall.

How can one stay thin, and be healthy?

A starch based diet is the solution!

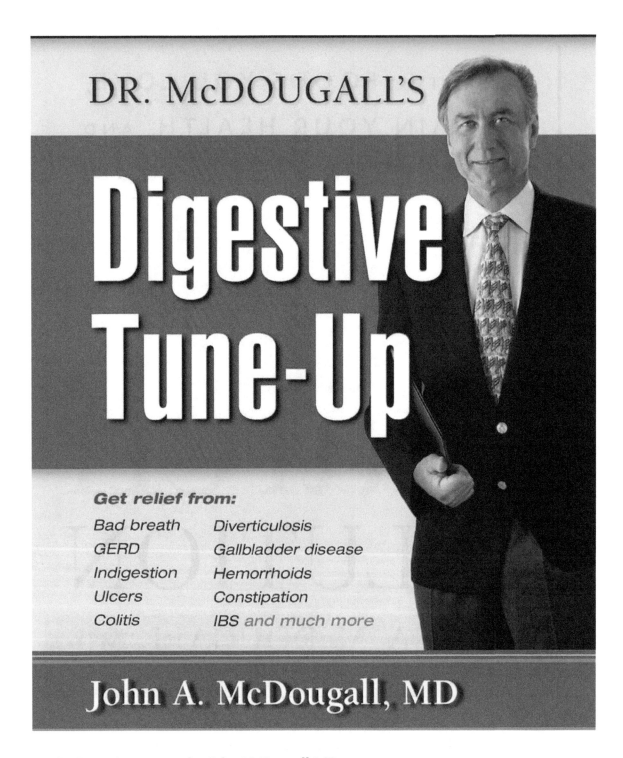

Fig 1-3: Digestive tune up by John McDougall MD.

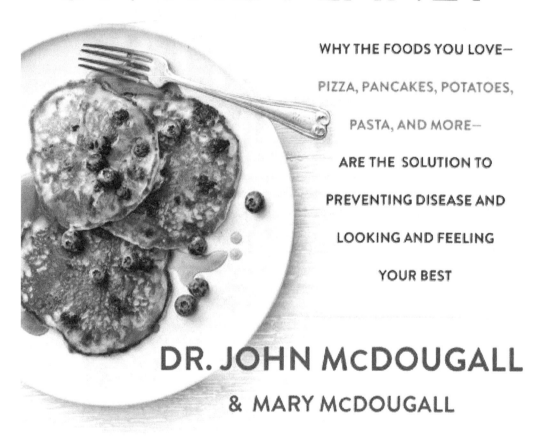

Fig 1-4: The Healthiest diet on the planet by Dr John McDougall & Mary McDougall.

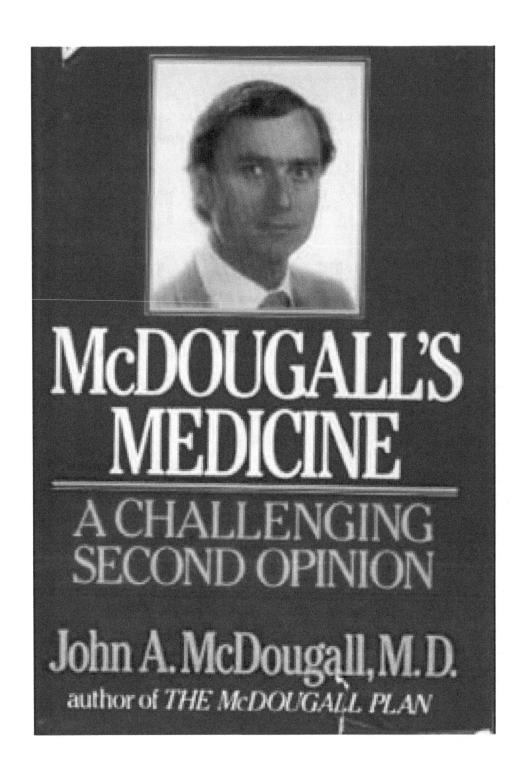

Fig 1-5: McDougall's medicine: a challenging second opinion by John McDougall MD.

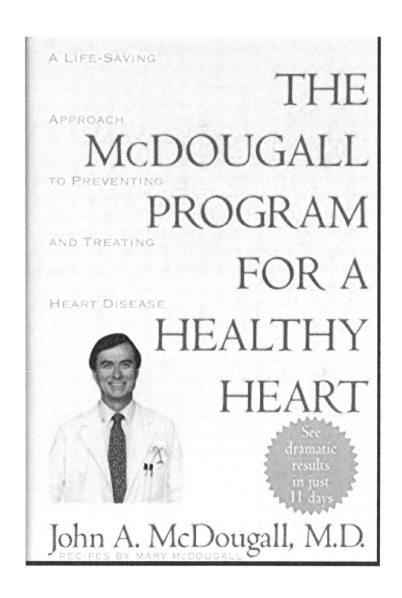

Fig 1-6: The McDougall program for a healthy heart by John McDougall MD, with recipes by Mary McDougall.

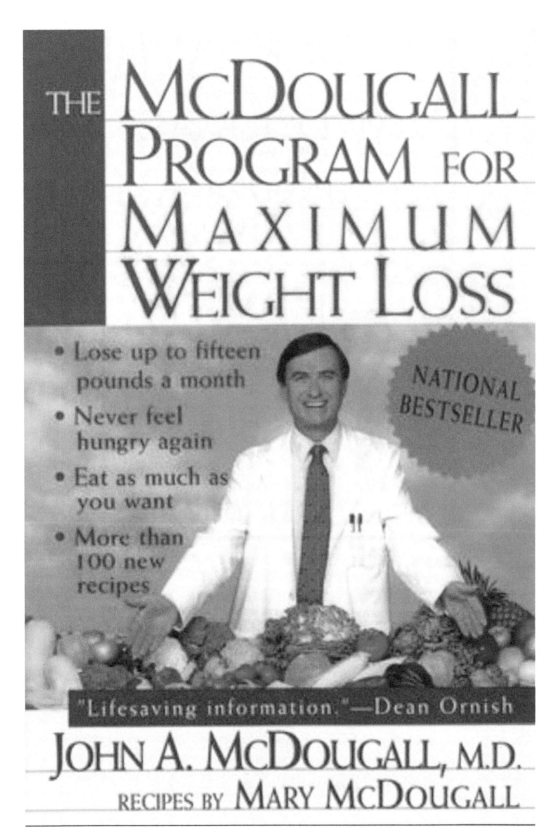

Fig 1-7: The McDougall program for maximum weight loss by John McDougall MD with recipes by Mary McDougall.

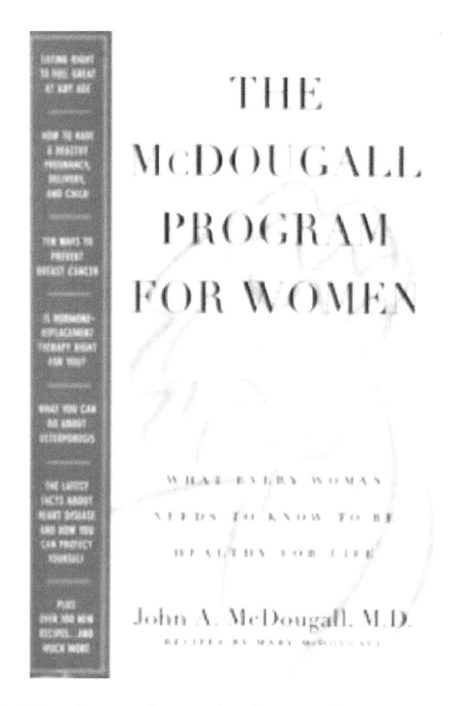

Fig 1-8: The McDougall program for women by John McDougall MD with recipes by Mary McDougall.

This book is a summary of Dr McDougall's nutrition and medical work.

Chapters will consist almost entirely of Dr McDougall's work.
Keywords for important concepts and for **reference papers** will be bold in black ink.

Titles of Dr McDougall's videos will be bold in blue ink.

All videos reviewed are from Dr McDougall's you tube channel.

This book only includes brief summaries.

If you are interested in a topic, you should go to Dr McDougall's you tube channel, and watch the entire video.

In general, things in **bold red ink will tend to be bad,** such as related to more disease.

In general, things in green will be good, such as related to treatments.

Occasionally, Dr Rogers, will add some clarifying comments which will be set apart by **[ ] brackets.**

Also, Dr Rogers will sometimes add some of his medical drawings to help explain pathophysiology.

Dr John McDougall is a genius who dramatically improved outcomes for many common diseases,

and who taught the world how to understand disease, from a nutrition and epidemiology perspective.

"A genius is someone who transforms a field"   – DK Simonton (1948-), expert on geniuses.

"When a true genius appears in the world, you man know him by this sign, that **the duncies are**

all in confederacy against him."   - Jonathan Swift (1667-1745)

"Scholars are those who have read in books, but thinkers, men of genius, world enlighteners, and reformers of mankind are those who have read directly in the book of the world….

All truths pass through three phases. First: ridiculed. Second: violently opposed. Third: accepted as self-evident...

Talent works for money and fame. Genius works for motives less easy to determine...

Talent hits a target no one else can hit. Genius hits a target no one else can see."
                  - Arthur Schopenhauer (1788-1860) .

"The world is always ready to receive **talent** with open arms. Very often it does not know what to do with genius. Talent is a docile creature. It bows its head meekly while the world slips the collar over it... It draws its load cheerfully and is patient of the bit and the whip.

But genius is always impatient of its harness; its wild blood makes it hard to train."

- Oliver Wendell Holmes Sr (1809-1894)

"All the greatest men are maniacs. They are possessed by a mania which drives them forward towards their goal.

The great scientists, philosophers, religious leaders - all maniacs.

What else but a blind singleness of purpose could have kept them in the groove of purpose.

Mania... is as priceless as genius."

- Ian Fleming (1908-1964), James Bond author.

"Every great work is the fruit of patience, perseverance and concentration - during months and years-upon one specific subject.

He who wants to discover a new truth must be capable of the strictest abstinence and renunciation.

 The ideal case would be that of a scientist who during this period of mental incubation, would pay no heed to any thought that is extraneous to his problem...

If he possesses this capacity to remain incessantly absorbed by one subject, he will be able to multiply his strength."

- Santiago Ramon y Cajal.

Chapter 2. **<u>Who is John McDougall?</u>**

John McDougall is the greatest doctor who ever lived, because he cured more patients than anyone else.

John McDougall was born in 1947 in the USA, to a humble, modest Scots-Irish family. He was very close with his parents. He died in 2024 at 77 years old.

As a freshman in college, John McDougall was fat, and a cigarette smoker. When he was 18 year old, he had a stroke, with paralysis of the left side of his body. He made a near complete recovery from the stroke, other than mild, left body residual weakness. The stroke motivated him to decide to go to medical school.

Dr McDougall became the greatest doctor who has ever lived.

His nickname became **Dr Potato.** Quite a story. An Irishman teaching the world that potatos are the best food in the world; that if he was only allowed to eat one food, it would be the potato.

His wife, and the love of his life, was Mary McDougall. They met when he was a medical student and she was a nurse in the 1960's.

Dr McDougall did his internship (first year of residency training) in Hawaii in 1972. As will quickly become clear, Dr McDougall is the doctor who fought for you.

I have fought the good fight, I have finished the race, I have kept the faith.

- 2 Timothy 4:7.

"I respond to emails from patients, and I used to respond to snail mail letters; because otherwise I'm as lonely as the Maytag repairman, because my patients get well." - Dr John McDougall.

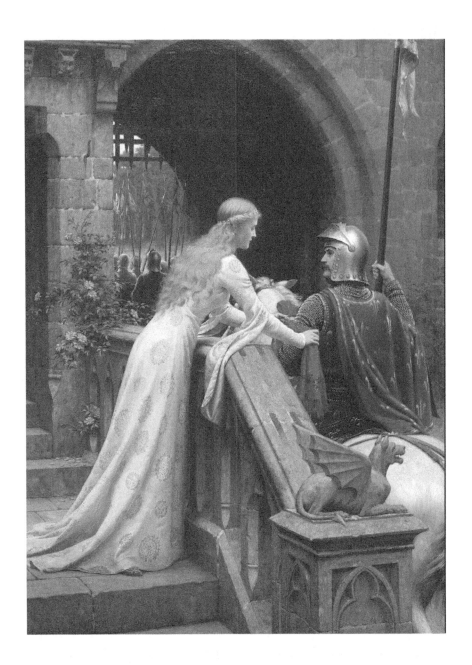

Fig 2-1: **God Speed!** by Edmund Leighton, 1900, public domain. Analogous to John & Mary. John and Mary rings a bell. Perhaps we should name a university "John & Mary," and dedicate it to nutrition and health?

The 1ˢᵗ priority of the medical system is NOT to help the patients. The 1ˢᵗ priority of the system is to make money.

Doctors are NOT obligated to really try to help the patients. Doctors are simply required to provide the STANDARD OF CARE. On the surface of it, the "standard of care" sounds like a great idea; something to live up to.

In reality, the standard of care means "drug based medicine," for the lowest common denominator. Lots of patients are drug addicts, intoxicated, unconscious, demented, etc. In order for a treatment to be "standard" for all patients, it has to be something that does not require the patient to do anything. because lots of patients are unable to do anything.

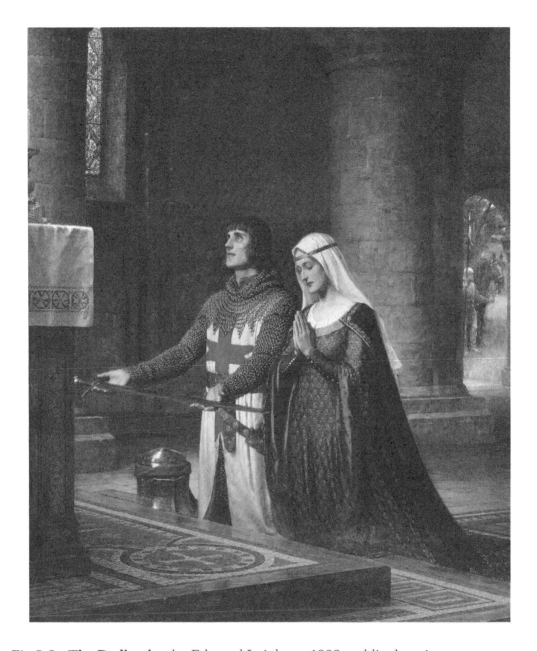

Fig 2-2: **The Dedication** by Edmund Leighton, 1908, public domain.

In reality, the standard of care is a sort of "animal" medicine. Ie. one could give a pill to a dog, or do a surgery on a dog. One could put a dog into a CAT scanner. Animal medicine is high tech & low intellect.

It's actually a much more sophisticated thing to have a conversation about the causes of a disease; and how a patient can change their diet and behavior to get a better outcome. Only humans can do that. This empowers the patient. Patient empowerment is low tech & high intellect.

Naive people think that artificial intelligence is going to improve medicine. Yeah right. Who do you think is going to write the AI programs? The drug companies! Of course. Gee, I wonder what they're gonna say? Perhaps, something like, "Prescribe more drugs. Especially the ones still under patent, that generate more profit."

21

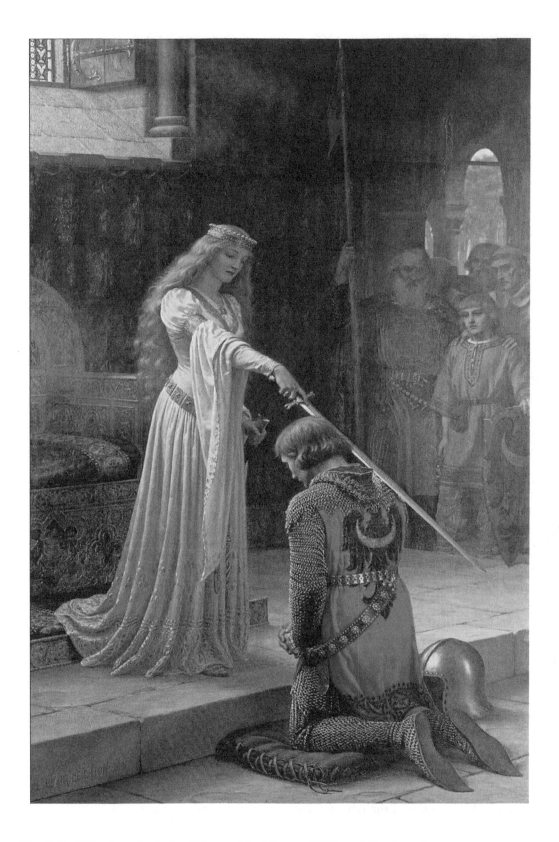

Fig 2-3: **The Accolade** by Edmund Leighton, 1901, public domain.

Who's got the money? The **drug companies**, of course. But it's not just them. The surgical **device manufacturers** bill for a lot. The **makers of machines** like CAT scanners & MRI machines are big business. The **for profit hospital corporations** are big business. Even the insurance companies are in on it, as the next story in McDougall's life will show.

McDougall noticed that low fat vegan diet almost always can cure heart disease (coronary artery atherosclerosis). John knew that he could teach the patients his starch based, low fat vegan diet in about one week; for fee of about $4,000; and almost all of them would be cured, if they actually followed the diet.

In comparison, coronary artery stents billed about $20,000 a piece, and coronary artery bypass graft (CABG) surgery billed for $100,000 (including operating room & surgical ICU fees). And the diet works MUCH BETTER. The diet actually cures the patient. Stents and CABG can help relieve anginal pain, but do not have a significant effect for preventing myocardial infarction or improving mortality.

Sounds great! Sounds like the insurance companies would love this! Like they would save money by having to pay less for patient cardiac care. Sounds like a sure deal. A walk in the park.

But that's not what happened. The insurance companies gave him the run around. They said that the education empowerment approach required too much cooperation on the part of the patient. McDougall thought this sounded like a weasel excuse.

The typical patient doesn't realize that the medical system considers them to be a bunch of morons. Many of them are morons, but the more motivated, intelligent ones should have the option of diet & lifestyle treatment.

"There's always a good reason, and then there's the real reason" – Thomas Carlyle ((1795-1881))

So, McDougall kept pushing to see what was the real reason that the insurance companies would not take the deal. Finally, an insider told him. **The bigger the payouts, the higher the insurance companies can set their premiums. The insurance companies are in on it too. They profit by overcharging the patients!**

How sad is that? **All of big money is against the patient:** big pharma, big hospital corporations, device manufacturers, imaging machine manufacturers, AND the insurance companies! They all want to rip off the patient. None of them wants to cure the patient.

"A patient cured is a customer lost!" – anonymous. Curing patients is bad for business!

The poor pathetic patient doesn't have much of a chance.

Now, do you think the other doctors at McDougall's hospital would celebrate his efforts? No! **They would NEVER send him a patient at St Helena hospital in California!**

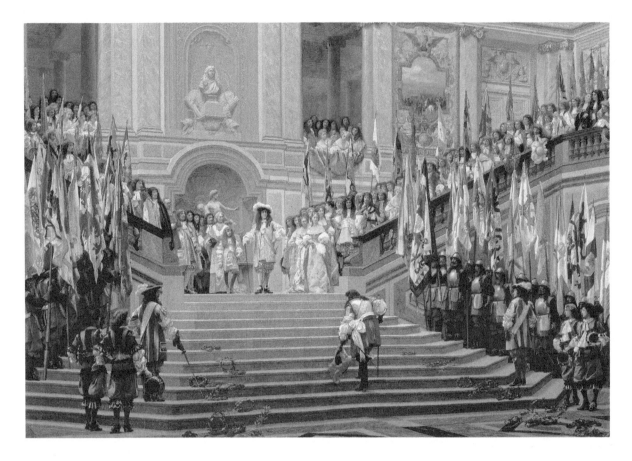

Fig 2-4: **Reception at the court of Versailles** by Jean Leon Gerome, 1878, public domain. This painting sums up what it was like for Dr McDougall to teach the low fat vegan diet to a sceptical health care system and population. To be a low fat vegan, one must be nonconformist.

"If one is interested in the relations between fields which according to customary academic divisions, belong to different departments, then he will not be welcomed as a builder of bridges, as he might have expected, but will rather be regarded by both sides as an outsider and troublesome intruder." - Rudolf Carnap (1891-1970).

The other doctors knew McDougall's methods were working. They could see that when patients went for followup coronary artery arteriograms or leg arteriograms, that the patients had improved. The other doctors would go to McDougall for advice about their own problems, and the problems of their family members.

Other low fat vegan doctors have had this same experience, like Dr Caldwell Esselstyn, and myself. In fact, Dr Esselstyn, had to use legal pressure to get his hospital, the Cleveland Clinic, to allow him to have an education empowerment clinic at the hospital.

In 1980, a citizen group in Hawaii was trying to get a law passed that women with breast cancer would be informed that mastectomy did not provide better outcomes than lumpectomy. This is because the horse is usually already out of the barn; ie. the patient usually already has micro metastases elsewhere, that will determine survival.

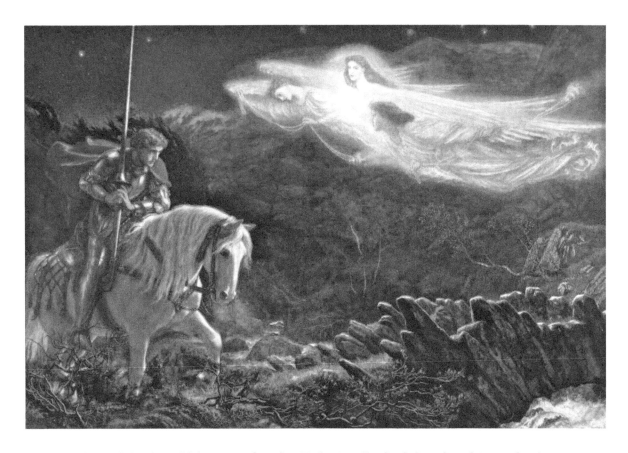

Fig 2-5: **Sir Galahad and his quest for the Holy Grail** which has the ultimate healing powers by Arthur Hughes, 1870, public domain. Dr McDougall and his quest to find the Holy Grail of healing. He found it! The Mcdougall diet! Low fat, whole foods, 100% vegan, with no oils.

McDougall helped to get the law passed. Did they throw a ticker tape parade for him? No! The **medical malpractice insurance at that time REFUSED TO RENEW HIS MALPRACTICE INSURANCE! They tried to put McDougall out of business. To bankrupt him.**

McDougall had to go bare (not have malpral insurance) for the next two years. Ouch!

Notice the pattern. When a doctor breaks out of the "standard of care" mode, the system attacks them.

Try to see it from big money's perspective. They designed the current system. They are making BILLIONS of dollars from it. They are like the biggest gang in the world of organized crime drug dealers. To them, a doctor is like a street corner drug dealer.

Do you think the leader of a drug dealing gang is going to let some little, street corner, drug seller change the system; so that they make less money? No way! They are going to kick his butt, and teach him a lesson, so that he learns to shut his mouth.

That's a big part of why doctors are so conformist. If they just **match the ill to the pill, and**

send the bill; then they make money, and they can't get into trouble. Even if the patient has a terrible outcome (as they so often do); even if the patient dies prematurely (as they so often do); it "doesn't matter."

As long as the doctor followed the standard of care, they are protected from a malpractice charge. If they educate & empower the patient, they don't get paid for it. And, they are at risk to get sued, if they did not prescribe the standard drug.

It takes a lot of time to explain stuff to patients. Every hospital and clinic in the Western world has a bean counter. The bean counters are in charge of the "assembly line." All the bean counters care about is through put; **how many billing codes are generated each day.**

If a doctor tries a McDougall approach to helping patients, they will soon get a warning from the bean counter, that goes something like this:

"You know Dr Diet, you are only seeing 15 patients a day. The other doctors in the clinic are seeing 30 patients a day. You are not pulling your weight. This is unfair to the other doctors. This is unfair to the clinic as a whole. You need to see 30 patients a day, or we're gonna have to let you go."

Dr Diet has limited choices. #1. he can stop teaching vegan diet; but then he will feel like a hypocrite, and be sad. #2. he can continue to educate the patients, but still see 30 patients a day; but then he will go home at 10 pm at night; become sleep deprived, and burn out. #3. He can start his own diet therapy based clinic; but it is very difficult to generate money when doing this.

McDougall chose option #3, and he made it work. His book sales also helped him to make a salary.

However, Dr John McDougall is a genius. He graduated first in his medical school class. Dr McDougall knows the medical literature of nutrition and health better than anyone in the world. He is famous for having a near photographic memory.

When someone asks him a question, he can routinely spout off the scientific paper that answers the question. He summarizes the nutrition literature, and his thoughts on it in his world famous medical newsletter which is available free at Dr McDougall dot com. He has all his newsletter editions memorized, and can give the specific dates of topic issues when asked.

The average doctor is not going to be able to pull this off. Ignorance is bliss.

Doctors are not taught Nutrition, Epidemiology & Toxicology (NET) in medical school or residency. But NET are the three most important topics for understanding disease and helping patients.

After finishing medical school and residency, doctors are exhausted, and typically heavily in debt with student loans. They usually apply for jobs in private practice, and hope to become partners in a group.

The groups often work them into the ground the first couple of years with lots of weekend, and night call. Simultaneously, they typically get married, and have a child; so they are overworked and sleep deprived. They want to make partner with their medical group so that they will make more money and have better job security.

The last thing in the world they would want to do is to piss off the system by trying to change anything! That's why there is ALMOST ZERO innovation in medicine.

Whenever a doctor tries to be creative and improve something, they get smacked down like whack-a-mole.

Now, I know what the average patient is thinking; that the doctor could go to a continuing medical education (CME) course, and learn about Nutrition, Epidemiology & Toxicology(NET). Yeah right.

Typical male doctor is a workaholic. His wife is glad for the money coming in, but she feels neglected with him working all the time. She reminds him that she hasn't gone on vacation in a long time, but her friends husbands take their wives on vacation & spend more time with their wives.

It's a subtle hint that he'd better take her on vacation soon, or he's going to be sold into slavery, and become a divorce mule.

So, they go to Florida for a CME course. In the morning he signs the attendance sheet for the CME course, so he can get his CME credits; then he goes with his wife and kids to pool or the beach for the rest of the day.

Even if he went to the lectures, it doesn't matter. Who do you think funds these CME meetings? The drug companies & the device manufacturers. What do they teach? That doctors should prescribe more drugs, perform more surgeries, and order more CAT scans! Duh!

That's why doctors like John McDougall are so rare. There's no money in it! And the system doesn't thank you. It kicks your ass! The system doesn't love you. It hates you!

"No one is more hated than he who tells the truth" – Plato (428-347 bc).

"In times of universal deceit, speaking the truth is a revolutionary act" – George Orwell, (1903-1950).

Now naive people might say, "Well, what about outcomes? If Dr McDougall is getting such great outcomes, why wouldn't people see that; and send him more patients; so he makes more money?"

On the one hand, Dr McDougall has thousands of patients with great outcomes. On the other hand, conventional medicine NEVER CURES THE COMMON CHRONIC DISEASES!

That's why they're called "chronic." It's like Dante's "Divine Comedy," when Dante and Virgil approach the gates of hell: the sign says "abandon hope, all ye who enter."

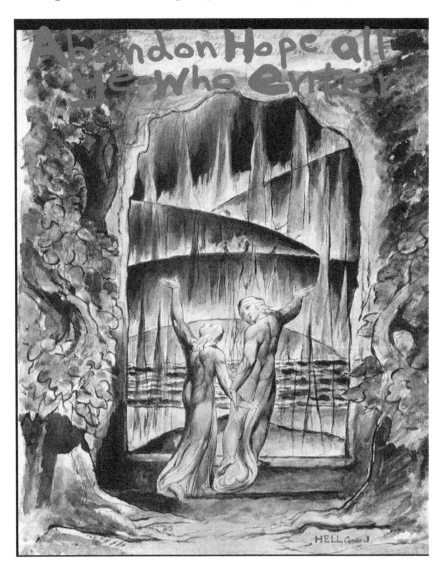

Fig 2-6: **"Gates of Hell seen by Dante and Virgil"** by William Blake, 1810, public domain. Conventional medicine for chronic disease says essentially the same thing, **"Abandon hope (of a cure) all ye who enter."**

Conventional medicine admits that it can NEVER cure the common chronic diseases like hypertension, diabetes, and atherosclerosis.

28

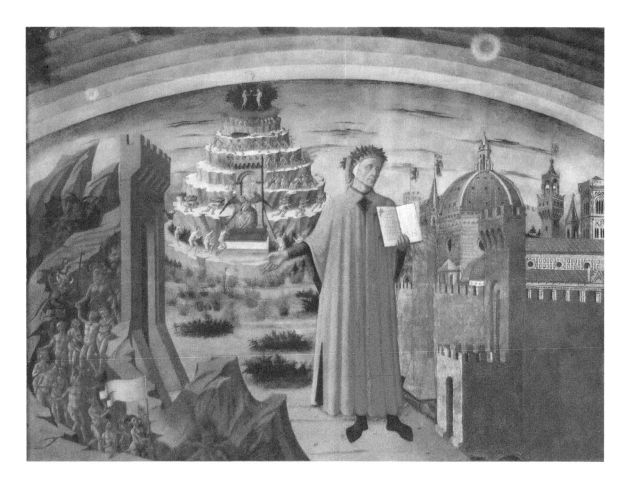

Fig 2-7: **Dante with Divine Comedy** by Domenico di Michelino, 1465, public domain.

Dante stands between Inferno and Florence. Purgatory behind him, Take your pick: SAD diet,

drugs & pills is the ticket to health hell. High fat vegan diet is the path to health purgatory. Low

fat vegan is the best chance to get to health heaven.

That's why conventional medical hospitals and clinics do NOT keep track of outcomes. They do
keep track of billing codes and "productivity," because that's how they make their money.

What happens to the patient is IRRELEVANT. As long as the standard of care was provided,
they can't get sued.

Patients are considered irrelevant, because they don't have any money. All a patient can do is
say, "Thank you." They usually don't even pay for their care directly. The insurance company
usually pays the bill.

If they started tracking outcomes and comparing them, someone would start using the
McDougall Method, and get much better results. That would be embarrassing to the the

healthcare system. That's why they never track outcomes!

Isn't it obvious. The doctors are beholden to the standard of care, and to the insurance companies.

Where does the standard of care come from? The big name research, university hospitals write the standard of care. Their doctors run the clinical trials to find out which drugs work best. In order to get promoted, and get a higher salary, they have to publish research papers.

In order to do a research project, they need grant money. Well, who's got the money? The drug companies! Are the drug companies a bunch of medical monks who want the best for everyone, and willing themselves to live in monastic poverty?

No! The drug bosses are a bunch of badass businessmen. One way or another, they are going to get their money, and anyone who gets in their way is going to get their ass kicked.

So, when the Ivy league medical professor goes a begging for money to big pharma, they essentially tell him: "Make our drug look good; or else!"

So what is the Ivy professor going to do. If he kisses the drug company's ass, he gets grant money, and publications, and a job promotion, and more salary money, and his wife is happy.

If he publishes a study saying that the company's new drug doesn't work, then he gets ZERO grant money. The drug company might even pressure the university to fire the professor. This happens all the time.

Eg. When T Colin Campbell published papers showing that animal protein was harmful to health, they tried to fire him from Cornell; and he was lucky to have tenure, that protected him from being fired.

I have a friend, who is a molecular biologist, and his friend published a paper showing that high fructose corn syrup (HFCS) is often contaminated with mercury. Did his university celebrate this brilliant discovery? No! The processed food company pressured the university to fire him; and they did!

This is what the system wants: patients "hooked" on drugs for life. The motto of the healthcare system is "Just say YES to DRUGS!"

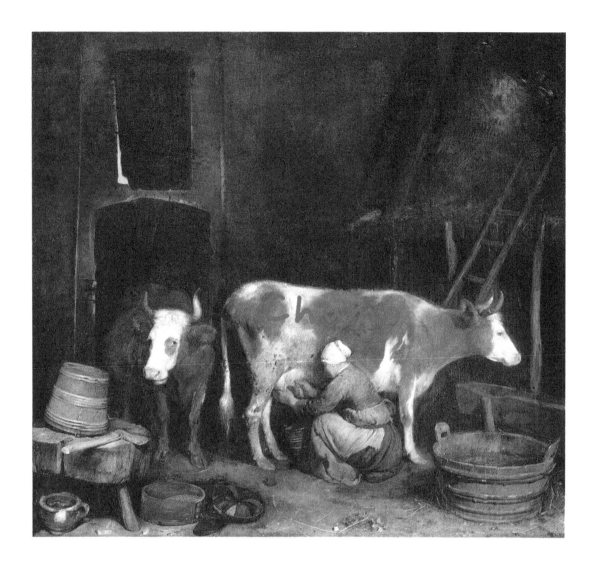

Fig 2-8: **Patients taking "medications" for diseases that could easily be cured by low fat vegan diet, are chumps who get milked like cows, by the system every day.** Painting is "Maid milking cow" by Gehard ter Borch, 1654, public domain.

So, now you know why Dr McDougall is such a rare bird. First, he had to be very curious and smart to learn all this stuff; second, he had to love the patients to we willing to fight for them. Third, he had to be very brave to fight the system which does not tolerate nonconformity.

A colleague said to Dr McDougall, "Why can't you just talk about nutrition? Why do you criticize stuff that other doctors do, like mastectomy, stents and CABG?"

Dr McDougall said, "I took an oath to protect the patients. I did not take an oath to protect the financial interests of the medical industry."

A lot of people did not like Dr McDougall: industries like big food, fast food, big meat, big dairy, big pharma, cancer industry, insurance companies, diabetes industry, hypertension industry, stent industry, olive oil promotion club, omega 3 promotion club, etc.

In their eyes, this Dr McDougall character is some kind of a crazy Don Quixote; who thinks he's trying to save the world, with all this knight errant tom foolery.

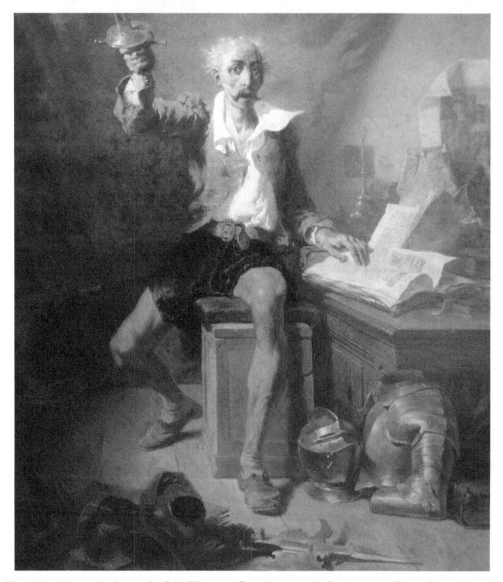

Fig 2-9: **Don Quixote in his library** [getting carried away reading about Knights, Damsels & chivalry] by Celestin Nanteuil, 1873, public domain. Don Quixote knows he's right, and decides to get on his high horse, and fight for the truth, as a knight errant.

Like Don Quixote, Dr Mcougall decides he's gonna fight for the little guy.

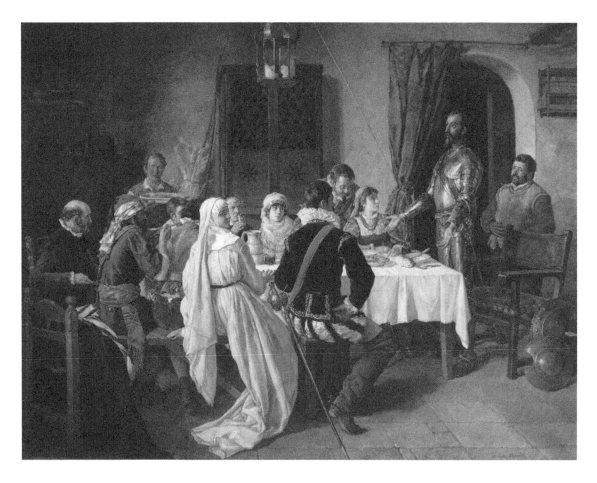

Fig 2-10: **Don Quixote's speech** by Manuel Garcia Hispaleto, 1884, public domain.

Like Don Quixote, Dr McDougall announces to his colleagues and friends that he is going to be a different kind of doctor; a doctor who empowers the patient, by educating them about diet.

When Dr McDougall told his residency director about his plans in 1976, the reply was that he was making a big mistake. That all he had to do was follow the standard of care, drug dealing playbook, and he would keep a big stable of patients, and make good money.

Instead he was going to teach the vegan diet. His chief resident said, "Who would want that? Your patients will probably be a bunch of bums and hippies. No one is going to pay you to talk about the vegan diet. You and your family might starve to death."

Who knows what'll happen with all the nutrition education stuff. The residency director worried that Dr McDougall, and his family, might go bankrupt, and starve.

It became obvious to me that diet was the most important thing for health...Given this new found knowledge about diet and health it became impossible for me to practice medicine the way I'd been taught. **I would be a different kind of doctor.** One who would empower my patients with the knowledge and ability to truly be well. - Dr John McDougall from Digestive tuneup, p. 4.

Dr McDougall knew the medical literature better than anyone else in the world. Like Don Quixote, Dr McDougall's library was burned down in a fire. I'm sure it was just a conincidence, and had nothing to do with all his billion dollar foes.

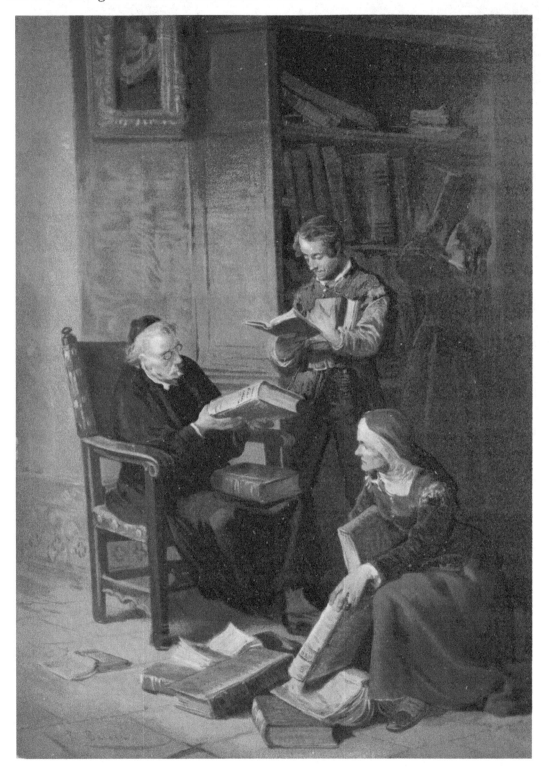

Fig 2-11: **The priest and the barber go to burn Don Quixote's library** by Ricardo Balaca, 1880, public domain.

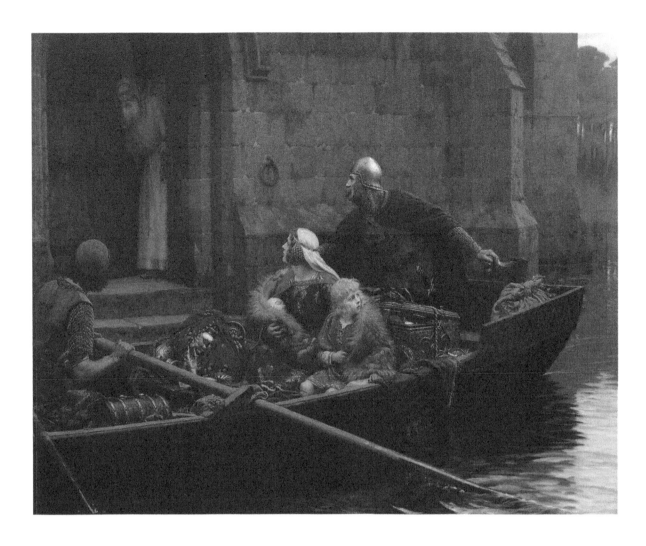

Fig 2-12: **In Time of Peril** by Edmund Leighton, 1897, public domain. Dr Mcdougall and his family had to flee their home, after the fires.

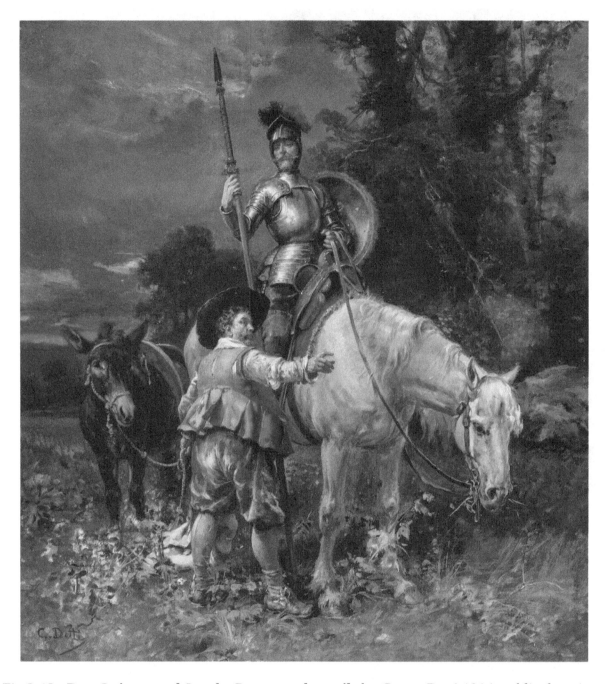

Fig 2-13: **Don Quixote and Sancho Panza on the trails** by Cesare Detti 1914, public domain.

I can imagine one of Dr McDougall's friends, like perhaps Doug Lisle, saying something like,

"You know John, you might not want to piss off the insurance companies or the big food companies or the surgeons. They have a lot of money. They could make things difficult for you."

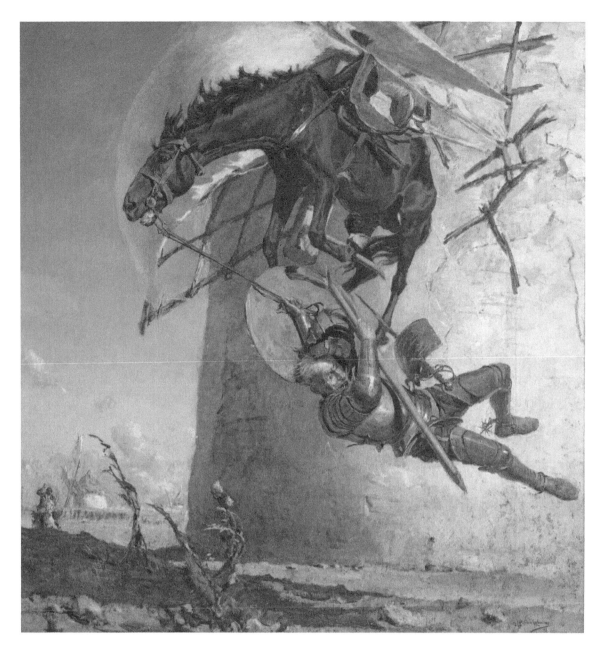

Fig 2-14: **Don Quixote fights the windmill** by Jose Moreno Carbonero, 1900, public domain.

To industry, and many of colleagues, Dr McDougall seemed like some sort of ridiculous, Don Quixote, taking on giants, who could so easily crush him.

Reminds me of the St Augustine (354 - 430 AD) quote: "Wrong is wrong, even if everyone is doing it. Right is right, even if no one is doing it."

And the Dostoevsky quote: "The goal of human life is more than just staying alive; the goal is finding something to live for.

God and the devil are fighting for the heart of men.

Sometimes – even if he has to do it alone –

and his conduct seems to be crazy;

 a man must set an example;

and so draw men's souls out of their solitude,

and spur them to some act of brotherly love;

that the great idea may not die...

We are all responsible for everyone, and I am more responsible than anyone else."
- Fyodor Dostoevsky (1821-1881).

Dr McDougall hung around with people that the medical industrial complex hates like Peter Gotzsche who said, "In medicine, there are VERY FEW people who like to hear the truth.

Screening mammography does more harm than good, and should be abolished.

There are lots of asymptomatic "cancers" in the breast and thyroid that are overtreated.

Psychiatry is one of the worse fields in medicine, and does far more harm than good.

Prescription drugs are the 3rd leading cause of death after MI & cancer."

On Wikipedia (July 2024), Dr McDougall is slandered. He is described as making "extreme dietary recommendations… that are not supported by evidence… of promoting a low fat fad diet… of **vegetarian extremism**… of being a **vegan zealot**… being out of touch with nutritional reality… of promoting a diet that is potentially too high in fiber, and too low in protein, calcium, iron, and omega 3 fats."

In essence, **Wikipedia describes the greatest doctor in the history of the world as a quack.** That is the thanks Dr McDougall gets for trying to help the proles.

If you read the medical textbooks, and the medical literature, you will see that **doctors who create profitable procedures are celebrated as heroes.** Eg. Andreas Gruntzig, inventor of coronary artery balloon angioplasty is heralded as a great hero of medicine and science. Wikipedia celebrates him as "opening up the therapeutic arterial highway" of the coronary

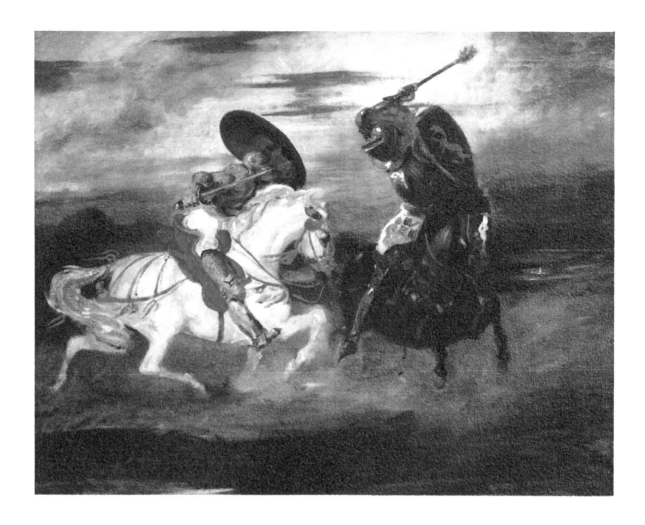

Fig 2-15: **Fighting Knights** by Eugene Delacroix, 1824, public domain. Dr McDougall debating the Paleo Keto Atkins crowd.

arteries. His USA medical center had an operating theater for him so that hundreds could watch him on TV perform coronary artery angioplasty in the early 1980's! They wanted to spread the procedure as quickly as possible.

The only problem is that coronary artery balloon angioplasty does NOT increase patient survival. The McDougall diet is proven to prevent coronary artery disease, and to save lives.

Why is Gruntzig celebrated as a hero, and McDougall called a quack? Because Gruntzig made billions of dollars for the medical system. McDougall taught the proles how to avoid needing the system.

I've gone through numerous **medical textbooks. I've never seen any of the nutrition doctors mentioned in those books** about the role of nutrition in preventing and treating disease.

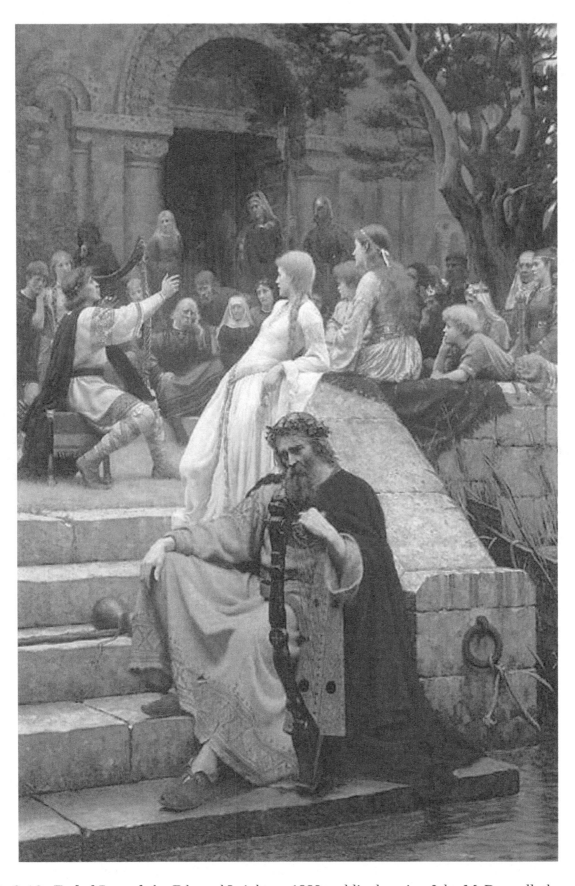

Fig 2-16: **Faded Laurels** by Edmund Leighton, 1889, public domain. John McDougall, the greatest doctor whoever lived, is ignored by medical textbooks, & shunned by big money media.

In his entire career, of 51 years, Dr McDougall was NEVER sued for medical malpractice. **Thousands of patients on the internet declare that Dr McDougall saved their lives!**

Dr McDougall also helped found the **American College of Lifestyle Medicine.**

Dr McDougall also got a law passed in **California** called **senate bill 380** which requires 11 medical schools to teach nutrition to medical students. And the bill also tells 500 hospitals in California that they are supposed to include nutrition as a topic in their noontime conferences.

"The most important thing in medicine is food." - John McDougall MD.

"The book, the college, the school of art, the institution of any kind, stop with the past...

This is good they say - let us hold by this. They pin me down. They look backward, not forward.

But genius looks forward...

Man hopes: genius creates…. "The **scholar** is that man who **must take up into himself all the ability of the time**, all the contributions of the **past**, all the hopes of the future... it is for you to know all...

Whoso would be a man must be a **nonconformist**. For **nonconformity** the world whips you with its displeasure… It is only when thy cannot answer your reasons that they wish to knock you down…

The best **argument** is not the accosting in front of the hostile premises, but the flanking them by a new generalization which incidentally disposes of them...

Colleges hate geniuses, just as convents hate saints…

Universities are of course hostile to geniuses, who seeing and using ways of their own, discredit the routine..

God offers to every mind its choice between truth and repose. Take which you please; you can never have both…

The office of the scholar is to cheer to raise and to guide men by showing them facts amidst appearances. He plies the slow unhonored and unpaid task of observation…

But he in his private observatory, cataloging obscure and nebulous stars of the human mind which as yet no man has thought of as such – watching days and months sometimes for for a few facts; correcting still his old records – must relinquish display and immediate fame.

In the long period of his preparation, he must betray often an ignorance and shiftlessness in popular arts, incurring the disdain of the able who shoulder him aside.

Long he must stammer in his speech; often forgo the living for the dead. Worse yet, he must accept – how often! - poverty and solitude. For the ease and pleasure of treading the old road, accepting the fashions the education the religion of society, he takes the cross of making his own…

and the position of virtual hostility in which he seems to stand to society, and especially educated society. For all this loss and scorn, what offset?

He is to find consolation in exercising the highest function ns of human nature. He is one who raises himself from private considerations, and breathes and lives on public and illustrious thoughts.

He is the world's eye.

He is the world's heart.

He is to resist the vulgar prosperity that retrogrades ever to barbarism, by preserving and communicating heroic sentiments, noble biographies, melodious verse and the conclusions of history…

these he shall receive and impart…

These being his functions it becomes him to feel all confidence in himself and to defer never to the popular cry. He and he only knows the world."

- Ralph Waldo Emerson (1803-1882).

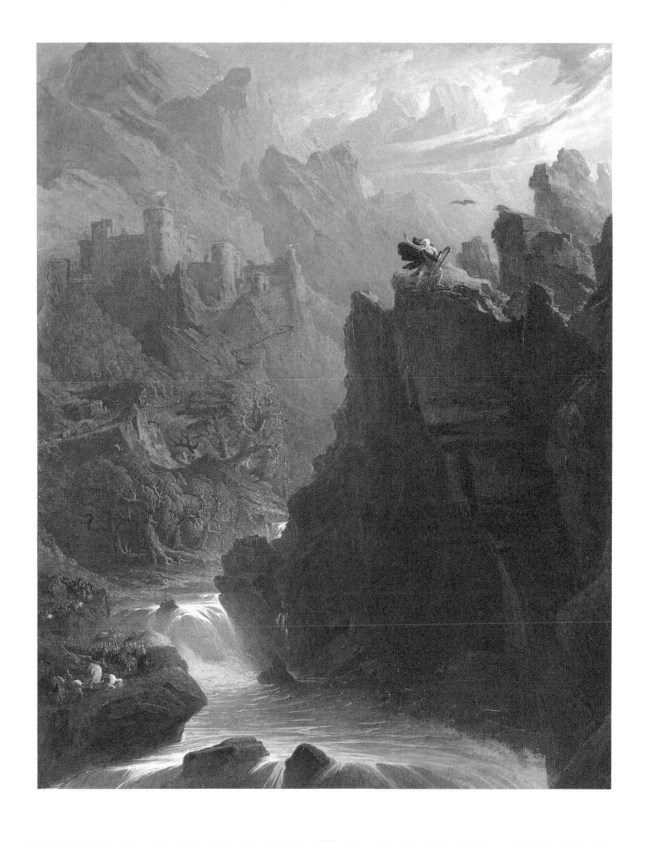

Fig 2-17: **The Bard** by John Martin, 1817, public domain. Dr John McDougall, like John the Baptist, cries out in the wilderness, to whoever will listen. The secret of health is Starch. Starch is the solution to your health problems. I've found the Holy Grail of health. It's starch!

Chapter 3 **Who is the greatest doctor ever?**

In a private practice hospital, the BEST doctor is the one who makes the most money for the hospital.

When I was in private practice, I started out working as an imaging guided surgeon (interventional radiologist). I had a patient with multiple problems, including a cardiac problem.

The cardiac problem was a simple one. I had rotated through interventional cardiology during my fellowship at Brigham & Women's hospital of Harvard. I figured the private practice cardiologist would quickly, successfully complete his procedure.

But he didn't. The cardiologist screwed up the case, and the patient had a bad outcome. I said to one of my colleagues, "that cardiologist screwed up the case. It was an easy case."

My colleague said, "Stop it! You can never criticize cardiology. Cardiology brings more money to this hospital, than all the other departments.

That guy you were talking about, he brings more money to this hospital than anyone else. If the hospital administration ever hears you talking about him, they will come after you, not him!"

Me, "Oh. So that's how it works in private practice? The best doctor is the one who makes the most money for the hospital."

I obviously belong in a research university, but I had comeback to my hometown to help out with my mother's care, who was suffering from metastatic cancer. I missed the university health care system.

In university research hospitals, the best doctor is the one who publishes the most papers. When I first heard of a doctor who published 100 papers, I was impressed.

Then I heard of doctors who had published 200, 300, 400, even 500 or more papers. I was astounded. I thought to myself, "What geniuses they must be! I can't wait to meet them. It will be so interesting to hear them talk. I'm going to learn so much. This is great!"

Then I started to meet some of them. My training has taken me through some of the most famous research universities in the world, and I have friends at many of the other places, who tell me about the star researchers there.

When I was at Northwestern, a chairman job was open, and a big shot from John Hopkins cam for an interview. His resume was over 50 pages long. He was going to give an audition lecture. I was excited to see it.

During his audition lecture he proved that he was a low IQ blowhard. He didn't say a single interesting thing. It was all socially sophisticated BS, that I already knew as a first year resident.

I remembered my second year of medical school, when I had a great professor in pathology: Dr Kirshenbaum. He was so clever. He took complex subjects, and made everything clear and logical. Using his approach to study pathology, I won the award as best medical student out of 333 in pathology.

I told my dad about Dr Kirshenbaum. My dad said, you will remember him for the rest of your life. I said, "Oh yeah, right. There's going to be lots of great professors."

My dad, who was a psychiatrist, said, "No. Most of the big name doctors are phonies. They get promoted for their social skills, not their knowledge. I can count on one hand the number of geniuses I've met in medicine."

I didn't believe it. As a medical student, I was cranking through the pathology, biochemistry, pharmacology books, and I was in awe of the authors. I dreamed that someday, maybe I could be a professor at one of the great research universities, and write a great textbook like these research stars had done.

I ran into more research "stars," and kept seeing the same pattern, they were mostly medical hierarchy ladder climbers, no thinkers. They would become section chiefs in their specialties, and then force all their underlings to put their name on every research paper that came out of the department.

Here's a typical experience; I ran into an imaging guided surgery colleague, just a little older than me, who had trained at a famous research university. I told him that I liked the textbook from that university.

He said, "Yeah, thanks."

I said, "What do you mean, thanks?"

He said, "I wrote that textbook."

I said, "BS! That book was just written a few years ago. You were just a fellow."

He said, "Yes. The boss over there pressured me to write the book. I had to do it. I needed a recommendation letter from him. I'm glad you liked the book, but I really didn't know that much. I was just a fellow. The book just seems good, because all the other books on that topic suck."

I later realized that he was correct.

I did occasionally meet some real geniuses, and a new pattern emerged. When a doctor becomes great, they start wanting to improve things, to change things.

The establishment made their reputations with the old way. The establishment makes money off the old way. They tend to hate the innovator.

The chairman of Mass General, Harvard radiology hated the smartest doctor on his staff, and vice versa.

The best imaging guided surgeons at other hospitals were often seen as wild men, and bad mouthed by the old timers.

My dad was right. After finishing medical school, and residency, I had met a lot of good people, but I had only had personally met 5 great teachers. I had seen others from other universities, but they were rare, and often in trouble with their departments.

Many of the great ones are known for being kind of eccentric, and are more interested in their discoveries, and inventions, than in money.

The other bizarre thing I learned is that the medical system does NOT care about the chronic disease patients. It just likes to "match the ill to the pill, and send a bill." The equivalent in dentistry is "drill em, fill em & bill em."

Strange as it sounds, it's more profitable to keep the patient sick, than to cure them.

In conventional healthcare, no one tracks outcomes. They can't do that! If they compared patient outcomes, then some wiseguy would come along, and start treating people with the low fat vegan diet, and he would have better outcomes than anyone else.

That cannot be allowed!

Instead, most Western hospitals focus on "productivity" which is a euphemism for "money." How many billing codes are generated per day. How many per each employee. Every Western hospital has LOTS of bean counters, but no one who feeding beans to the patients.

Well, what do patients want? Patients want to be cured!

Who do patients think is the best doctor?

47

The doctor who can cure the most patients!

What are the most common diseases?

The chronic Western diseases like obesity, hypertension, diabetes, atherosclerosis, abdominal pressure syndrome, etc.

Why are they called "chronic?"

Because conventional medicine can NEVER cure them!

But Dr McDougall cures these diseases all the time? Yes, he does. That's why he's the best doctor, ever.

But Walter Kempner MD saw 19,000 patients, and had incredible records of cures.

Yes, he did. And, Dr McDougall said that Dr Kempner was probably the best doctor who ever lived.

However, then Dr McDougall came along. Dr McDougall saw 12,000 patients in person. So, it might seem at first that Dr Kempner cured more patients.

However, Dr McDougall cured many tens of thousands of patients more, maybe hundreds of thousands more by his books like Starch solution & Gastrointestinal tuneup; and by his free newsletter(the best one) at Dr McDougall dot com; by his tele-health clinic; and by his internet videos that have been viewed by millions of people.

"Tele-health is the medicine of the 21st century." - Dr John McDougall.

Dr John McDougall has cured more patients than any doctor who ever lived. The McDougall diet routinely cures people of obesity, hypertension, type 2 diabetes, coronary artery disease, and often of autoimmune disease, and many other diseases.

There's no other doctor who's even close.

Dr McDougall, at his website, has pages and pages of testimonials from patients cured by his advice, and the McDougall diet.

There's no other doctor who's even close.

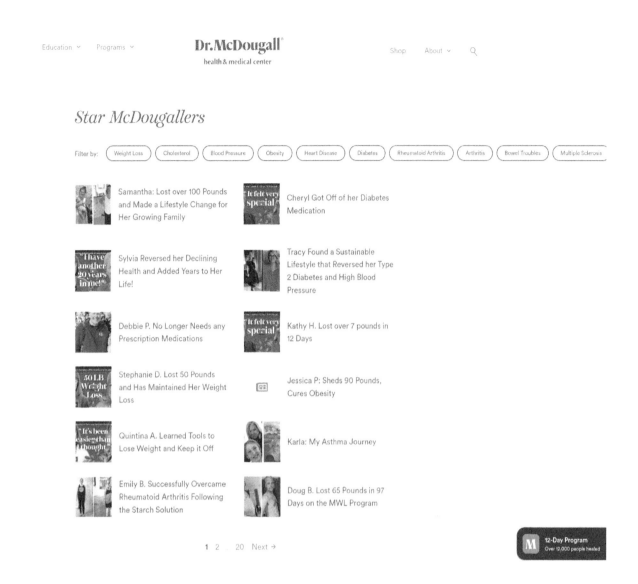

Fig 3-1: A sampling of the numerous patients cured by Dr McDougall's advice, and the McDougall diet from Dr McDougall's website, Dr McDougall dot com.

No other doctor has that. Conventional medicine NEVER cures these common, chronic diseases. The patients have to take pills for the rest of their lives, and the pills tend to not work so well, so they usually end up going for surgeries, that also tend to not work so well. Then the patient ends up prematurely fat, sick, stupid, broke, and dead.

Dr John McDougall has cured far more patients than any doctor who ever lived. That's why Dr John McDougall is the greatest doctor who ever lived.

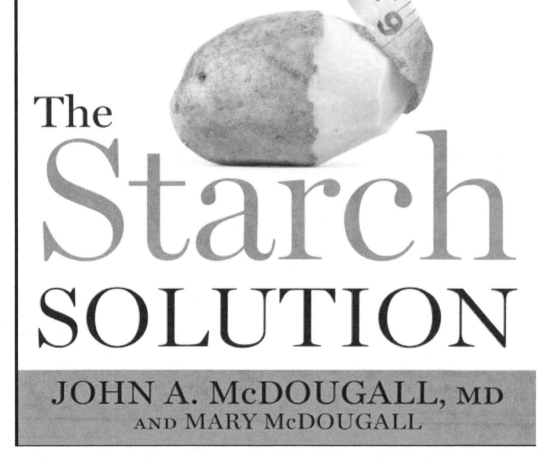

EAT THE FOODS YOU LOVE,
REGAIN YOUR HEALTH, AND
LOSE THE WEIGHT FOR GOOD!

The
Starch
SOLUTION

JOHN A. McDOUGALL, MD
AND MARY McDOUGALL

Fig 3-2: "The Starch Solution" is considered by many, myself included, to be Dr McDougall's best book.

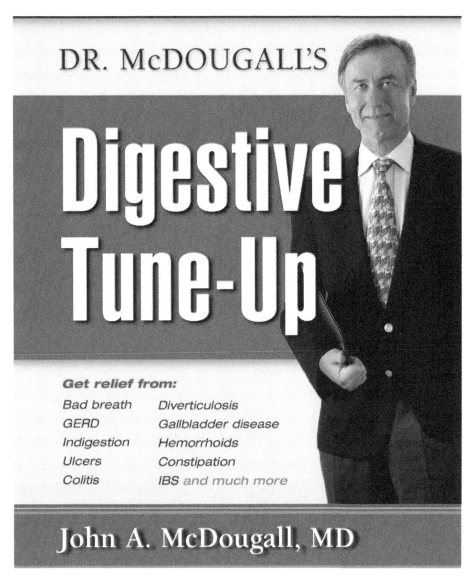

Fig 3-3: Gastrointestinal Tune-up by John McDougall MD is a great book. Very easy to read. Nice illustrations. Explains the common abdominal diseases.

Dr McDougall wrote a monthly health & nutrition newsletter from 1986 to 2017. The article index for the McDougall newsletter is at DrMcDougall.com.

Chapter 4. **_Dr McDougall's medical achievements_**

What did Dr McDougall do?

He provided a systematic, rational way to understand health.

He figured out the most important thing that anyone could know about health: that people should eat a starch based, plant based diet.

He figured out that this is the most important variable for determining whether people will be thin and healthy, or fat and sick.

*********AO (Academic Orgasm) alert!**********

Starch is what you do!

Epidemiology is how you know it's true!

Dr McDougall figured this out. I made it into a rhyme, so that it wil be easier to remember. It seems so simple, yet there is more wisdom in those two sentences, than in all the medical school books.

Those are the two greatest secrets of health.

If a person eats a starch based, whole food, vegan diet, then they almost certainly will be thin with no type 2 diabetes, and a good blood pressure, and clean coronary arteries, and a relatively low risk of cancer.

Starch is what you do! Epidemiology is how you know it's true.

"**Simplicity** has always been held to be a mark of truth; it is also a mark of genius. Students and learned persons of all sorts and every age, aim as a rule at acquiring information rather than insight.
Information is only a means of insight, and of little value in itself.

For the man who studies to gain insight, books and studies are merely rungs of the ladder on which he climbs to the summit of wisdom. Thinking in search of insight is what makes a man a philosopher.

 The object of science is to recognize the many in the one, to perceive the rules in any given example and not to go on counting up facts ad infinitum." - Arthur Schopenhauer (1788-1860) .

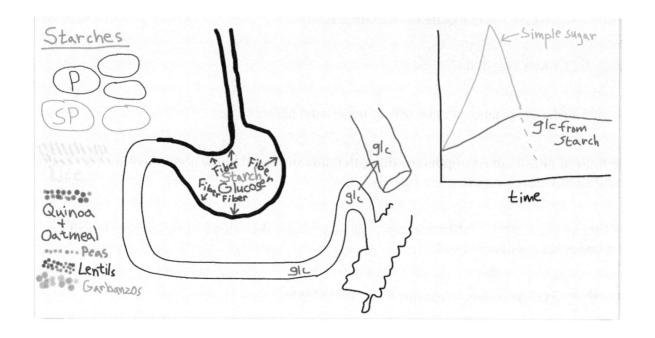

Fig 4-1: Starch is low caloric density, so it stretches the stomach with relatively few calories; Stretching the stomach provides early satisfaction of hunger.

Then the starch goes into the small bowel. Starch is a polymer (means bunch of connected molecules) of glucose wrapped in fiber.

The small bowel enzymes need time to separate the glucose from the fiber. This gives starch the "effect" of being like a slow, gradual release energy "pill."

Glucose is slowly absorbed from the gut to the blood. This keeps the blood glucose level in a good range for a prolonged amount of time. This satisfies hunger for a prolonged amount of time.

This satisfies hunger with the fewest calories, so starch eating populations are thin.

"Starch is the best food to satisfy hunger" – Dr John McDougall.

Eat starch

Why?

Dr McDougall studied the starch based diet from multiple angles, and saw that the benefits were empirically and logically consistent.

Starches = best food to satisfy hunger. Starches taste good, are called "comfort foods."

Starches are almost always low fat, (except for soy), store well, are cheap, are the healthiest food, and tend to not store up toxic chemicals.

Potatos & sweet potatos are complete foods, except for vit B12 .

Grains & legumes are almost complete except for vitamins A & C.

Fruits and vegatables provide vitamins A & C.

Epidemiology shows that a starch based diet creates the healthiest populations.

Migration studies show that a starch based, plant based diet works best.

Research by Kempner, Burkitt, Blankenhorn, Burkitt, Pritikin, Campbell, Swank & others shows that a plant based works best.

Longevity studies show that a starch based diet works best. Seventh Day Adventists are the longest lived, well documented population.

The oldest living person in recorded history is 122 years.

The average vegan 7th day Adventist male lives to about 85 and female to about 89 years old.

"The Bible suggests that adults often lived into their 70's and sometimes into their 80's."
- John McDougall MD.

"Seventy years are given us. And some may even live to be eighty."
- Psalms 90:10.

Comparative anatomy supports a plant based diet. Humans have starch taste receptors in their mouth. Humans have flat teeth for grinding plants.

The human jaw can partially go sideways for grinding food, unlike a carnivore cat which has a fixed forward bite, which makes it's bite much stronger. Humans have a long intestinal tract, like plant eating mammals. Humans don't make vitamin C, presumably because there is so much available in plant foods. Human hands are made for gathering plant foods, not for tearing flesh.

Starches were able to provide the necessary nutrients for brain development. It was not necessary to eat meat.

Military histories of Alexander the Great (356-323 bc), Julius Caesar, Gladiators & Genghis Kahn (1162-1227 ad) said they fought best with plant based diet = rice, wheat, and barley. The gladiators were called the "barley men," (hordearii = barley).

The bones of gladiators were analyzed, which indicated they ate a starch based diet. The Roman soldiers of Julius Caesar's legions complained when they had too much meat, because they said they preferred to eat grains before fighting.

During WW1 & WW2, the populations who had **rationing of meat and dairy,** had lower frequency of the Western diseases.

This also showed that the diet had a bigger effect on health, than did psychological stress. Ie. despite a lot of stress, they were still healthier, in terms of less atherosclerosis and autoimmune disease.

Marathon runners: Best runners are the Kenyans. They eat 80% of their calories from starch, especially maize. Ugali is corn meal molded into balls. Also bread, boiled rice, boiled porridge, cabbage, andbeans.

Carl Lewis the 9x olympic gold medalist followed the McDougall diet, and subsequently set the record for the 100 meter dash.

Paleontology studies show that a plant based, starch based diet works best. For example, the Egyptian mummies who ate rich diets had atherosclerosis, gallstones, and obesity.

Reference: Sutherland et al. Atherosclerosis across 4,000 years of human history: the Horus study of four ancient populations. Lancet, 2013, Apr 6; 381(9873):1211-22.

Dr McDougall's **personal experience** with himself, his family & his patients also showed that a starch based diet works best.

It's not exercise, because even the sedentary people who eat a low fat starch based diet are thin & healthy.

It's not genetic, because when thin healthy populations migrate to USA & change diet → they lose their health.

What are some examples of epidemiology to support a starch based diet?

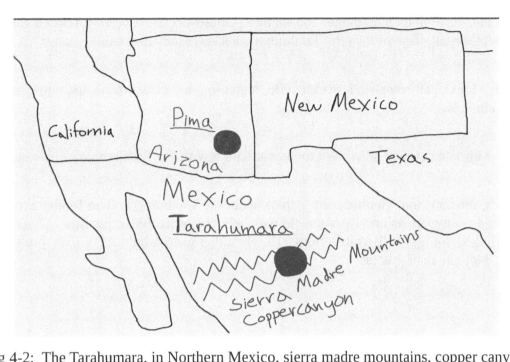

Fig 4-2: The Tarahumara, in Northern Mexico, sierra madre mountains, copper canyon area eat a starch based diet, especially corn, beans, squash, and local greens.

The PIMA were absorbed into Arizona after the Mexican American war in 1848. The PIMA now eat a SAD diet, and have the typical Western diseases. Ie. it's the diet, not the genetics.

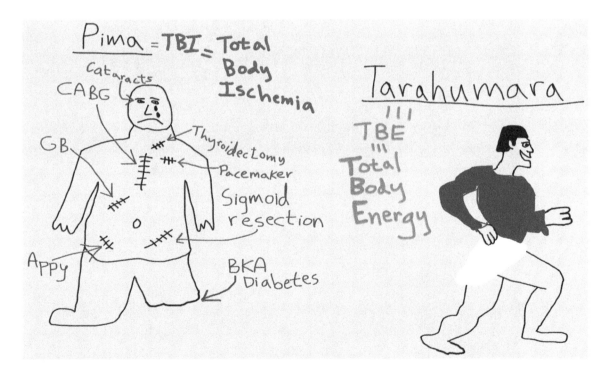

Fig 4-3: The PIMA are train wrecks of health with lots of obesity, hypertension, diabetes, atherosclerosis, gallstones, etc.

The Tarahumara are world famous ultramarathoners. Tarahumara can run over 100 miles in two days. Famous American runners have gone to visit the Tarahumara.

Ruth Heidrich Phd, champion marathoner and triathlete, multi-decade survivor of breast cancer, patient of Dr McDougall, went to visit the Tarahumara, and says they are real.

Reference: Dr McDougall newsletter, march 2006, high protein diets harmful, and unnecessary for endurance athletes.

Scott Jurek, star ultramarathoner, also went to visit and train with the Tarahumara.

William Connor, the nutrition scientist wrote papers about the Tarahumara. The Tarahumara are thin, and do not have hypertension. Even the old people have normal blood pressure. Their average total cholesterol was 136, triglycerides 115. Their diet was carbohydrate 75%, protein 13%, fat 12%. Not one man was fat.

Nathan Pritikin was so impressed by the endurance of the Tarahumara, that he patterned his diet after them. Christopher McDougall (not related to Dr McDougall, as far as I know) wrote a book about the running ability of the Tarahumara, called "Born to Run."

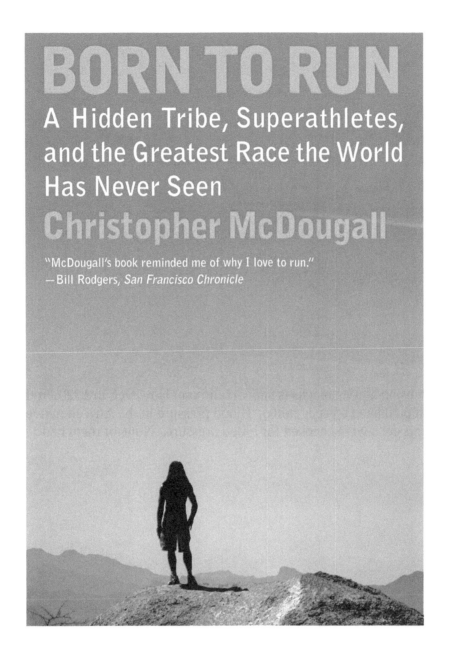

Fig 4-4: Born to run by Christopher McDougall (not related to Dr John McDougall, as far as I know) wrote about the amazing running endurance of the starch eating Tarahumara.

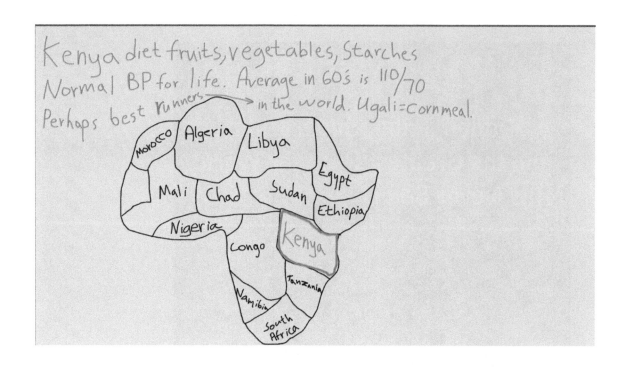

Kenya diet fruits, vegetables, Starches
Normal BP for life. Average in 60's is 110/70
Perhaps best runners → in the world. Ugali=Cornmeal.

Fig 4-5: In USA, hypertension among blacks is super common. However, in 1929, in the Lancet journal, Donnison published a paper called "Blood pressure in the African native," for which 1,800 hospital admissions were checked for blood pressure. None of them had hypertension!!!

Blood Pressure in the African Native. Its Bearing upon the Aetiology of Hyperpiesia and Arterio-Sclerosis.

Author(s) : Donnison, C. P.

Journal article : Lancet 1929 pp.6-7 pp. ref.7

Abstract : The investigations recorded in this paper were made on natives resident in a large reserve, that of S. Kavirondo in Kenya Colony, living in primitive conditions, that is conditions which have remained unchanged probably for centuries. Men only were examined, chiefly young men recruited for labour needs in various parts of the Colony; older men were seen when the author was on tour. The places of examination were at 5, 700 feet and down to 3, 500. It seems unlikely, he writes, that such altitudes could have any marked influence upon the blood pressure of the inhabitants. The ages were estimated. The instrument used was an aneroid sphygmomanometer by Down Bros. A series of 1, 000 examinations was made on apparently healthy natives ranging from 15 years to 70 or 80 years. [img 2T27311.tif]

Up to the 4th decade the figures for the two races approximately agree. After that the blood pressure, both systolic and diastolic, tends to come down in the African, whereas in the white races it continues to rise till the 8th decade.

The author spent over two years at a native hospital where about 1, 800 patients were admitted and thus had a good opportunity of recognizing pathological conditions which might be the result of high blood pressure. No case of raised blood pressure was encountered and never was a diagnosis of arteriosclerosis or chronic interstitial nephritis made. Hypertrophied hearts, without intrinsic cardiac disease, are very rarely met with in the African. In autopsies it has been noted that the African usually shows much less atheroma in the aorta than does an average European of the same age.

The results, then, of this investigation support the view that hyperpiesia and arteriosclerosis are diseases associated with civilization. Considering the causation of high blood pressure the author discusses the two main views, the toxaemic theory, and that of the over-responsive vaso-motor system, or mental stress theory; he favours the latter and concludes that differences in the evolution of the two races must be held responsible for the differences in the normal standards of blood pressure. A. G. B.

Fig 4-6: Donnison paper from Lancet journal in 1929 checked blood pressure of 1,800 hospital admissions in Kenya, and ZERO% had hypertension!!!

In Kenya, the population was eating a plant based diet, and ZERO% had hypertension. In USA, the majority of middle age and older blacks have hypertension. Hypertension is also super common in other populations in the USA.

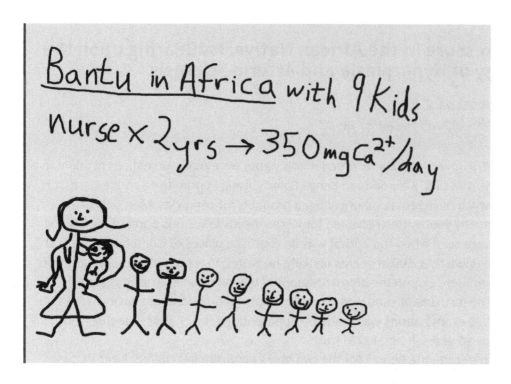

Fig 4-7: Osteoporosis in USA is NOT because of calcium deficiency. In the Bantu population of Africa, the woman typically have about 9 children, and nurse each one about 2-3 years.

The Bantu women have a very low calcium intake, but they do NOT have a problem with osteoporosis.

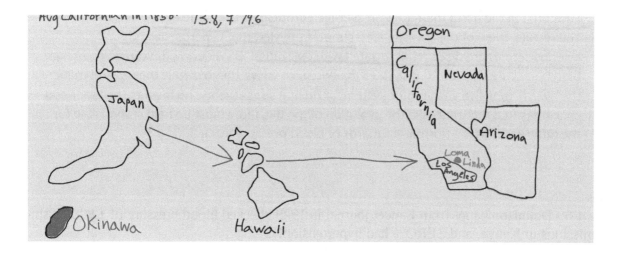

Fig 4-8: In Okinawa, where they ate lots of sweet potatos, they had 5x more centenarians than the USA. Many o fthe Okinawans were farmers, and they walked a lot. They had close families and communities. They venerated their ancestors. The also ate a lot of greens. Diet was about 80:10:10. Okinawan average age of death was 86 yo for women and 78 yo for men. They had very low risk of coronary artery disease or prostate cancer.

Japanese migrant studies showed progressively worse health as they moved from Japan to Hawaii, and then from Hawaii to USA, and westernized their diet. To westernize a diet means to eat more meat, dairy, and oil. The point is that the change in disease frequency is related to diet, not genetics.

Among the plant eating Seventh Day Adventists, the healthiest ones were the 100% vegans.

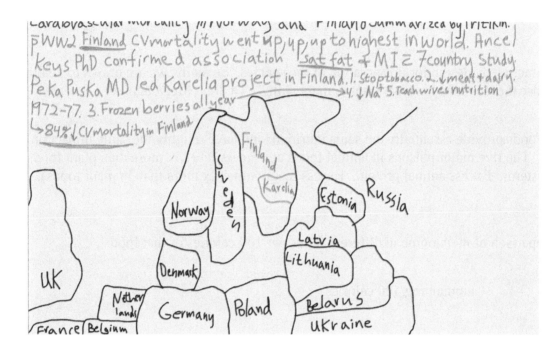

Fig 4-9: In the 1960's Finland was noted to have very high levels of cardiovascular mortality. In the 1970's, from 1972-1977, under the guidance of Pekka Puska MD, Phd, the Karelia province (the Karelia project), made a big effort to reduce their intake of meat and dairy, and of smoking tobacco, and to eat more plant foods. They had an incredible 84% drop in cardiovascular mortality.

This Karelia project outcome is one of the most incredible outcomes in all of medical research; just another example of the power of plant based diets.

Why did people start becoming so fat and sick? The industrial revolution of the 1800's brought more wealth. Meat and dairy became more available. In the 1900's electricity and refridgerators made it possible to store meat and dairy for longer amounts of time.

In Starch Solution, Dr McDougall uses epidemiology to answer the common concern of the public. The average, poorly informed American thinks that "starches make people fat."

Dr McDougall points out: Over a billion Asians mostly eat rice, and they are thin. In Peru, where they eat potatos, the people are thin. In Papua New Guinea where they eat sweet potatos the people are thin. **Reference: A**m j clin nutr 14;13-27, 1964. Total cholesterol average was 153mg/dl. Triglycerides level was 142 mg/100ml. No diabetes or gout were found.

Reference: J nutr sci vitaminol (Tokyo), 1981;27(4):319-31.

Dr McDougall also points out that these same starch eating populations have very low rates of diabetes, arthritis, constipation, gallstones, multiple sclerosis, heart disease, breast cancer, prostate cancer, colon cancer.

Dr McDougall says starch eating populations are healthier than other populations. Health is attractive.

"Health is attractive by design for preservation of the species. Sexually, we are drawn to healthy people, because those are the ones we want to mate with." - Dr John McDougall.

"All animal foods provide essentially the same nutrition, and have roughly the same impact on you health… The five major poisons in animal foods are excess fat (15x more than plant foods). Excess cholesterol. Excess animal protein. Excess methionine (4x more than in plant foods). Excess acid.

Here's a comparison of methionine in different foods per 100 calories of that food:

Food	amount mg/100 calories
potato	35 mg
rice	52 mg
Pinto beans	98 mg
whole eggs	251 mg
beef	250 mg
chicken	317 mg
Salmon	318 mg
egg whites	700 mg

" - Dr John McDougall.

A typical example of an animal food is salmon. Salmon is 50% fat, and 50% protein. That's a lot of fat, and a lot of protein! Animal foods do not have any fiber. Other than milk, there is hardly any carbohydrate in animal foods.

	Sat fat	Oil	Sodium	Tob	Fruits & vegetables	Dm	Htn	MI	Stroke	Impotence	Cancer
American	High	mod	Moderate 6 g/d	Low	Low	Mod to high	Mod to High	High	Moderate	High	High
E. Asian, Japan, Korea, China	Low	Low	High > 12 g/d	High	Moderate	Low	High	Low	High		Moderate
S. Asian, India	Low to mod (dairy)	High	High	Low	Low	High	High	High	mod	High	
Low fat, low sodium, vegan	Low	ZERO	Low	ZERO	High	ZERO	ZERO	ZERO	Very low	Very low	Very low

Fig 4-11: Low fat, starch based vegans have less hypertension, diabetes, myocardial infarction (heart attack), stroke, impotence, and cancer than other populations.

65

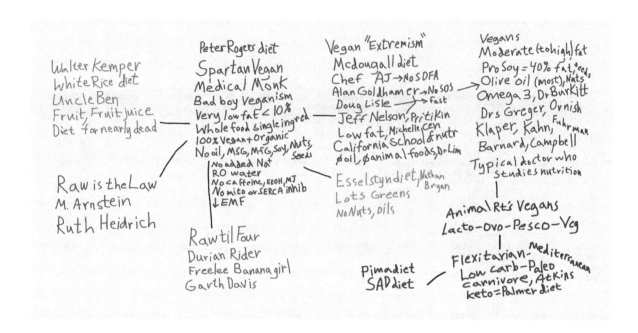

Fig 4-12: This chart compares many of the well known common diets. The McDougall diet is a low fat, starch based, vegan diet with no oils. Many persons have been heavily influenced by Dr McDougall. Dr McDougall's students comprise what I call the California school of nutrition.

I list Dr Esselstyn, adjacent, but separate, because he promotes large amount of greens for his high risk cardiac patients.

The McDougall diet is doable for the majority of the population. The USA population would dramatically improve it's health if it ate the McDougall diet.

Chapter 5. **McDougall's mentors**

Mentor #1. Denis Burkitt MD (1911-1993) = the FIBER man.

In 1971, Dr McDougall, as a senior resident in internal medicine, had a life changing experience at noontime conference.

Denis Burkitt MD was the visiting professor, giving a lecture about diet and disease. Denis Burkitt is an Irish surgeon, who did some of his training in England. He then went to Africa as a Christian missionary doctor. Dr Burkitt was in Uganda for about 17 years, and he almost never saw the common Western abdominal diseases.

By the way, Dr McDougall is Irish, & so is Dr John Kelly (author of stop feeding your cancer). & so is Peter Rogers (me), & I think T Colin Campbell Irish, Scottish or English. Kelly Turner Phd (author of Radical Remission, fiery red head, looks Irish), Michael Brownlee MD (name sounds Irish or Scottish, wrote best paper ever on diabetes). Durian Rider (Harvey Johnstone) (Australia, & Australians are often descendants of Irish "criminals" sent to Australia). Jeff Nelson is Scottish (I think). So those little places have produced some nutrition experts.

Denis Burkitt is the genius who figured out abdominal pressure syndrome. Burkitt lectured about how dietary fiber prevents abdominal pressure syndrome.

Fiber comes from plants. There is no fiber in meat and dairy. Processed foods tend to have very little fiber. Dietary fiber attracts water to the stool. This softens the stool. This prevents constipation. Denis Burkitt said that our ancestors routinely ate 100 grams of more of fiber per day. Nowadays, it is recommended that people try to eat around 50 grams of fiber per day, or more.

SAD (Standard American Diet) eaters eat only about 12 grams of fiber per day. Lack of fiber causes dry stools. When the stool is dry, in can form rock like stool balls called feca-liths = poop stones.

Fiber helps the body to remove excess estrogen and cholesterol by defecation.

It's normal to have a bowel movement 1 to 3x per day. In some can be normal to have only one BM per day. The key thing is that the stool is soft.

If a fecalith forms in the appendix, it is called an appendicolith. An appendicolith can obstruct the appendix where it connects to the cecum. The mucus glands in the distal appendix can continue secreting mucus. This will overstretch the appendix, until it bursts; spilling stool into the adjacent abdominal fat. That's appendicitis.

Plant eaters have soft bowel movements, like a cow patty. The soft stool stretches the rectum, and this causes a reflex contraction of the rectum, to evacuate the feces, almost effortlessly.

With SAD diet eaters, the stool is relatively dried out, and usually does not stretch the rectum that much. Lack of rectal stretch means lack of reflex rectal contraction; this leads to straining at defecation. Straining at defecation is called the Valsalva maneuver.

Valsalva maneuver generates back pressure into the abdomen. This back pressure pushes on the rectal veins causing rectal hemorrhoids.

The back pressure can be transmitted into the scrotum causing a varicocele (dilated veins) that can heat up the testicles, and lower testosterone levels and sperm counts.

Yes. It's true. Constipation can lead to infertility.

The Valsalva maneuver back pressure is also transmitted into the leg veins, and can cause varicose veins.

The Valsalva pressure also increases the risk of inguinal hernias, and anterior abdominal wall hernias (eg. periumbilical hernias).

The Valsalva pressure is also transmitted to the stomach, and this pushes on the diaphragm. The diaphragm separates the stomach from the chest. Valsalva pressure can widen the diaphragmatic hiatus (the hole in the diaphragm through which the esophagus passes to become the stomach).

The Valsalva pressure can then push the upper part of the stomach into the chest. This upward herniation of part of the stomach is called a hiatal hernia.

Hiatal hernias tend to lead to GastroEsophageal Reflux Disease (GERD). GERD tends to lead to inflammation of the lower esophagus which is called Barrett's esophagus. Barrett's esophagus is associated with increased risk of cancer.

Denis Burkitt said, "America is a constipated nation. If you have small bowel movements, you need large hospitals. If you have large bowel movements, then you only need small hospitals."

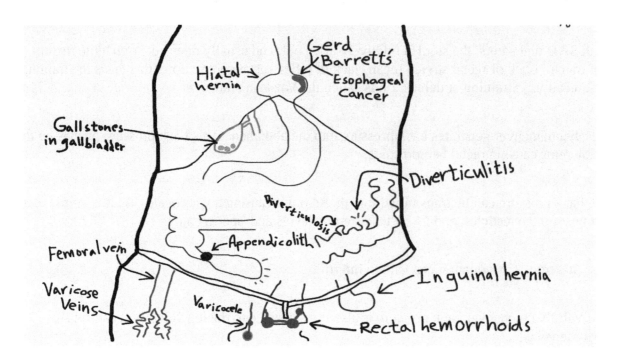

Fig 5-1: Abdominal pressure syndrome as described by Dr Denis Burkitt. Lack of fiber leads to dry stool. Dry stool leads to constipation, and straining (Valsalva maneuver) at defecation. Valsalva maneuver causes back pressure damage to multple parts of the abdomen, as illustrated here.

The only live interview video of Dr Burkitt on the internet was filmed by Dr McDougall and is viewable for free on you tube at Dr McDougall's you tube channel.

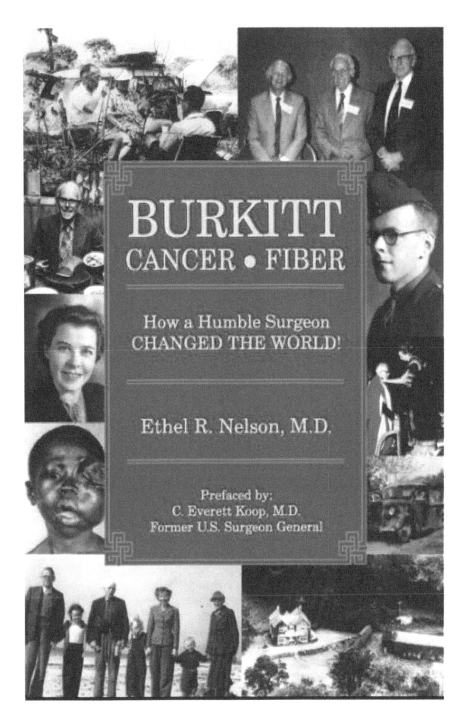

Fig 5-2: "Burkitt, cancer, fiber: how a humble surgeon changed the world" by Ethel Nelson MD is an excellent biography of Dr Denis Burkitt.

Reference: **Dr McDougall newsletter, January 2013, Denis Burkitt MD opened McDougall's eyes to diet and disease (includes video interview of Dr Burkitt from 1982).**

Dr McDougall wrote that: The key to big bowel movements is to increase amount of dietary fiber ... Dr Burkitt was the first doctor who ever told me that diet & health were directly related

That the foods we consume cause the majority of our most common chronic diseases

Burkitt (working in Uganda), noticed that meat & dairy eating westerners Americans only 4 oz stool/d. Plant eating Africans passed an average of 16 oz stool/d = 4x more stool!

Among plant eating Africans in Uganda → There was essentially no type 2 diabetes, obesity, appendicitis, diverticulitis, IBD (UC & Crohn's), dental caries, varicose veins, hemorrhoids, HH, or colon cancer!

Dr Burkitt only saw one case of gallstones in 20 years. He only saw1 heart attack from a judge recently returned home from London where he ate beef etc.

Denis Burkitt said "The frying pan, is something that you should give to your enemy...food should not be prepared in fat… our bodies are adapted to a stone age diet of roots & vegetables

Diseases can rarely be eliminated through early diagnosis or good treatment, but prevention can eliminate disease…

If people are constantly falling off a cliff, you could place ambulances under the cliff, or build a fence on top of the cliff, or build a fence on top of the cliff. We are placing too many ambulances under the cliff…

Western doctors are like poor plumbers. The treat an overflowing sink by trying to dry the floor. Somebody should teach them how to turn off the faucet" – Denis Burkitt.

If you want to learn more about Dennis Burkitt, you will find information at Dr McDougall's website, and here is a paper you might like: Denis Burkitt and the origins of the dietary fibre hypothesis by John Cummings, nutrition research reviews, 2018, 31, 1-15.

Mentor #2. **Walter Kempner MD** (1903-1997).

I was reading about Stephen Hawking the physicist with ALS, and his work didn't impress me. It seems to me that his basic assumptions were wrong. I said to myself, this guy is not a genius. Then I read that while he was in the hospital with ALS, that he seduced two nurses. Now, that's impressive! He must be a genius! I never dated a nurse. I asked out a nurse, and she told me that my vital signs were too abnormal for consideration.

However, even on his best days, Hawking can't hold a candle to Kempner.

Walter Kempner MD is the rock star of vegan world, likely for all time. He not only was king of the babes, and cured more patients than any other doctor of his time, but he also was a multi-millionaire. In fact, he was the biggest money maker at Duke university for years. Dr McDougall describes Walter Kempner as "the father of dietary therapy."

Dr Kempner used to go to the rice house every day, but he took 3 months off every summer! What a great job! The entire summer of 3 months off!

People from all over the world traveled to Durham to be treated by Dr Kempner with the rice diet. Before we get into all that, here's the story of Dr Kempner's origins.

Walter Kempner grew up in Germany. He graduated first in his medical school class. His mentor was Otto Warburg. Yes, that Otto Warburg. Discoverer of the Warburg effect; winner of the nobel prize in 1931.

Otto Warburg showed that when exposed to hypoxia, many cells will become dysfunctional or die, but some will transform into cancer cells. These cancer cells will burn glucose without oxygen; this is called anaerobic metabolism. This led to the metabolic theory of cancer, which is the best theory of cancer.

"The vast majority of cancer researchers believe that Otto Warburg was correct with his metabolic theory of cancer" – Dr McDougall from his online lecture "Does sugar feed cancer?"

Hans Krebs was also a student of Otto Warburg. Hans Krebs discovered the Kreb's cycle. Kreb's cycle runs in the mitochondrial matrix, and is also called the citric acid cycle or the tri-carboxylic acid cycle. Hans Krebs also won a nobel prize.

Walter Kemper deserved a nobel prize, they almost never give the mto nutrition doctors. Big money does not want the proles to find out about this nutrition stuff.

Kempner began the rice diet service at Duke in 1939. His two main groups of patients were kidney failure patients, and hypertension patients.[1] Many of his patients had what was called "malignant" hypertension, and were only expected to liver for about 6 months or less. Kempner saved many of them.

Doctors, like Frank Neelon, who worked with Kempner were amazed by the great outcomes. Frank Neelon said, "It was rather amazing. To go from the regular wards and clinic where patients are never cured of diabetes and hypertension, to then see Kempner's clinic where patients are routinely cured of these things."

Later on, many patients came to him for treatment of obesity.[2] Fat celebrities flocked to Durham including Elvis, Shelley Winters, Buddy Hackett, Dom DeLuise, Lorne Greene…

Kempner had a lot of experience treating kidney failure. Kempner had done research on kidney function.

Kempner knew that the main job of the kidney was to secrete nitrogen. Amino acids have nitrogen. There is no nitrogen in carbohydrates and fats. So Kempner decided to minimize protein intake in his kidney failure patients.

The kidney also excretes acid. Keeping the diet relatively alkaline, by avoiding animal foods, also helped to protect the kidneys.

Back in those days, there was no dialysis. Full blown kidney failure patients just died. Kempner's low protein, rice diet helped keep many of these patient alive for a long time.

Kempner's rice diet consisted of white rice (eg. Uncle Ben's rice), fruits, fruit juice, and table sugar. Kempner did add a multivitamin. Kempner carefully rinsed off the rice, and did what he could to minimize dietary sodium.

Now, why oh why, would he give sugar? Sugar has no nitrogen, so it's safe for kidney patients.

   Kempner knew that dietary **fat causes insulin resistance** → so he wanted to minimize dietary fat.

Kempner did NOT allow high fat foods like avocados and nuts.

———————————————

1 Kempner (1949) "Treatment of heart, kidney & hypertensive disease with rice diet" ann int med, 31 (5): 821-56

2 Kempner (1975) "Tx of massive obesity with rice reduction diet program." Analysis of 106 pts with at least 45 kg wt loss" arch int med, 135: 1575-1584.   avg wt loss 64 kg = 141 lbs. Also found on p. 516 of 570 in Kempner's "Scientific publications, vol 2."

The Kempner diet was about 93% carbohydrate, 3% fat, and 4% protein. Now that's a low fat diet!! See Dr Newborg's biography of Kempner, p. 120. The diet consisted of white rice, fruits, fruit juice, and a multivitamin. As the patients condition improved, vegetables could be added.

Thus, complex carbohydrates, (starch), provided at least 90% of the calories in the basic rice diet. Calories were restricted only when weight loss was also a goal.

For patients who were too thin, Kempner gave them table sugar so that he could add calories without adding sodium or protein.

"Carbohydrate food makes insulin work better." - Dr McDougall.

When Kempner's patients were studied quite closely, they did not have nutrient deficiencies.

The Kempner diet is quite boring, but it works. Dr McDougall described it as the "diet for the nearly dead." Many of Kempner's severe kidney failure and hypertension (eg. with systolics in the 200's) would have certainly died quickly, if it wasn't for the Kempner rice diet.

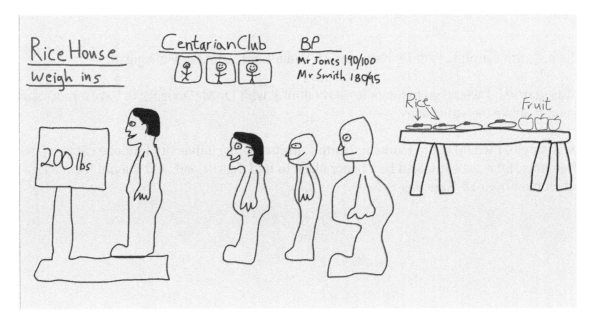

Fig 5-3: Weigh ins at Kempner's rice houses in Durham, North Carolina.

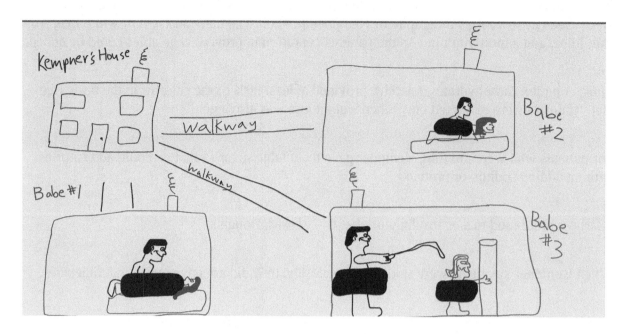

Fig 5-4: Walter Kempner was famous for being a lady's man. Dr Kempner was accused by some patients of whipping them with a riding crop when they did not comply with his rice diet. One patient claimed that Dr Kemper was boinking her, as a sort of sex slave for over a decade. Some say that she was an ex-girlfriend just trying to get more money from Kempner, after their breakup.

Kempner was tall and handsome. He never married. Kempner had a harem of girlfriends, paid for their college educations, and he bought houses for them, and connected the houses with walkways.

If I was a senior medical student, and I could only do one elective clinical rotation in nutritional therapy, where would I want to go?

Durham, North Carolina with Dr Kempner or Santa Rosa, with Dr McDougall.

If I was married, I would go to Santa Rosa [Podunk], with Dr McDougall, to have a more stable life, and to make the wife happy.

If I was single, I would got to Durham, North Carolina, Duke university [college campus], with Dr Kempner, b/because it would be a better place to find a girlfriend, and I could learn a lot about women from Dr Kempner.

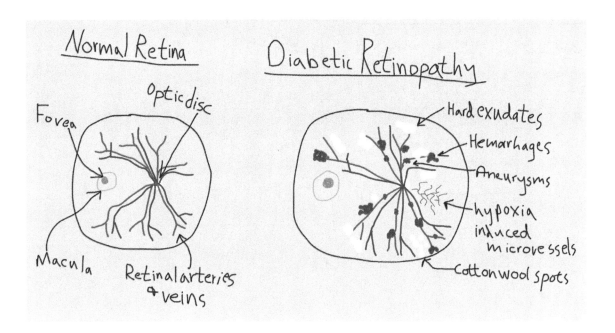

Fig 5-4: Kempner had incredible results for the eyes. In his patient notes, Dr Kempner had many patients who REVERSED the vascular disease in their eyes.

Kempner was most proud of hundreds of patients whose **retinal photographs** once scarred by hypertensive retinopathy & diabetic retinopathy, then **reversed**
to normal or near normal→ some with significant improvements in vision.

As far as patient was concerned it was like they guy in the Bible who said,

"I know not how he did it, but I was blind, and now I can see." Newborg's book about Dr Kempner, "Walter Kempner and the Rice Diet," p. 145. and Scientific publications vol 2, p 505, 516 of 570.

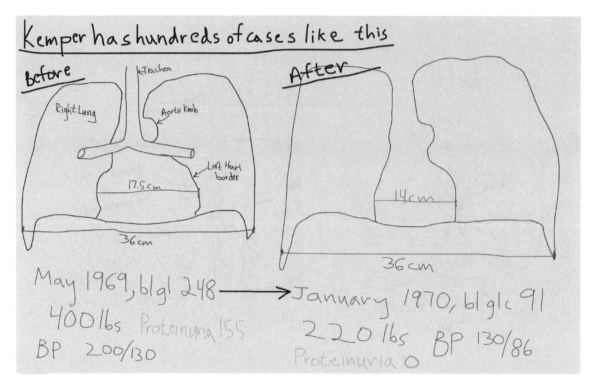

Fig 5-5: A typical patient from Dr Kempner's papers. Body weight decreased from 400 lbs to 220 lbs. BP decreased from 200/130 to 130/86. Blood glucose from 248 to 91. Proteinuria resolved. Cardiac size became normal on chest x-ray (CXR).

Many patients with rheumatoid arthritis and psoriasis also improved on the diet.

Dr McDougall, at his website, has Dr Kempner's publications available for free; including numerous photos of dramatic improvement in eye disease, chest disease, vascular disease, diabetes, hypertension, kidney disease, etc.

Dr McDougall said, "Do not even try to debate me, unless you have read the papers of Walter Kempner and Nathan Pritikin. If you haven't at least read that, then you're wasting my time."

If you go to Dr McDougall's website, you will find detailed description of Dr Kempner's work, and Dr Kempner's publications are also available.

If it was not for Dr McDougall, then Dr Kempner's work would have probably been lost. Dr McDougall is to Kempner's work, kind of like what Aquinas was to the work of Aristotle.

None of the great nutrition experts is in any of the standard medical textbooks: Zero for Drs Kempner, Burkitt, Swank, Esselstyn, McDougall, etc.

Dr McDougall also has Nathan Pritikin's legacy book available for free at his website.

Dr Kempner's work showed Dr McDougall just how POWERFUL dietary therapy can be.

Remember: conventional medicine NEVER cures hypertension, diabetes, and atherosclerosis. Kempner's diet easily, routinely cures these diseases.

VOLUME II
Radical Dietary Treatment of Vascular and Metabolic Disorders
Table of Contents

Foreword   1

1943

CASE REPORTS: *Discussion by Dr. Kempner*   3

1944

Kempner, Walter. *Treatment of kidney disease and hypertensive vascular disease with rice diet* [Poster presentation and talk, Chicago session of the annual meeting of the American Medical Association]   7

Kempner, Walter. *Treatment of kidney disease and hypertensive vascular disease with rice diet*   10

Kempner, Walter. *Treatment of kidney disease and hypertensive vascular disease with rice diet, II*   21

1945

Kempner, Walter. *Compensation of renal metabolic dysfunction: treatment of kidney disease and hypertensive vascular disease with rice diet, III. Part 1*   27

Kempner, Walter. *Compensation of renal metabolic dysfunction: treatment of kidney disease and hypertensive vascular disease with rice diet, III. Part 2*   59

1946

Kempner, Walter. *Some effects of the rice diet treatment of kidney disease and hypertension*   105

Fig 5-6: Table of contents for Dr Kempner's research papers at Dr McDougall's website. It's available for free.

79

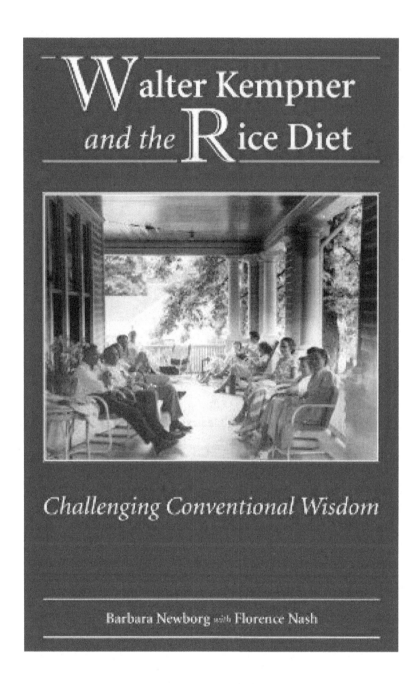

Fig 5-7: Biography of Walter Kempner & the story of the rice diet by Barbara Newborg. Dr Newborg was a physician who worked with Dr Kempner.

Like most female authors, she talks more about social stuff, than my autistic self would prefer, but it's still a great book, and she does go through the medical stuff like sodium management, disease reversals of EKG's, CXR's, retinal exams, weight loss, etc.

Dr McDougall newsletter, December 2013, Walter Kempner MD founder of the rice diet. Summarizes the work of Dr Walter Kempner with illustrations.

Dr McDougall newsletter, December 2014, arsenic in rice.

Arsenic in rice was discussed in the consumer reports magazine of Novermber 2012, and Nature magazine in October 2014.

Rice grown in California has about ½ the arsenic as rice from Louisiana. Because arsenic based insecticides were used, before being banned in 1988. Arsenic insecticides were used to kill boll weevils on cotton crops grown in southeastern USA: Arkansas, Georgia, Florida, Louisiana, Mississippi, Missouri, and Texas. Many of these same lands have been used to grow rice.

Similar scenarios have contaminated of other foods like apples and other crops.

There is less arsenic in white rice than in brown rice.

Animal foods are often worse. 90% of arsenic in USA diets comes from seafood.

Rice is the most common grain for human nutrition, and provides more than one fifth of calories to people worldwide.

Reference: Dr McDougall newsletter, Jan 2012, White rice works for most people.

Article says it's reasonable to eat white rice; that there was no significant benefit to eating brown rice.

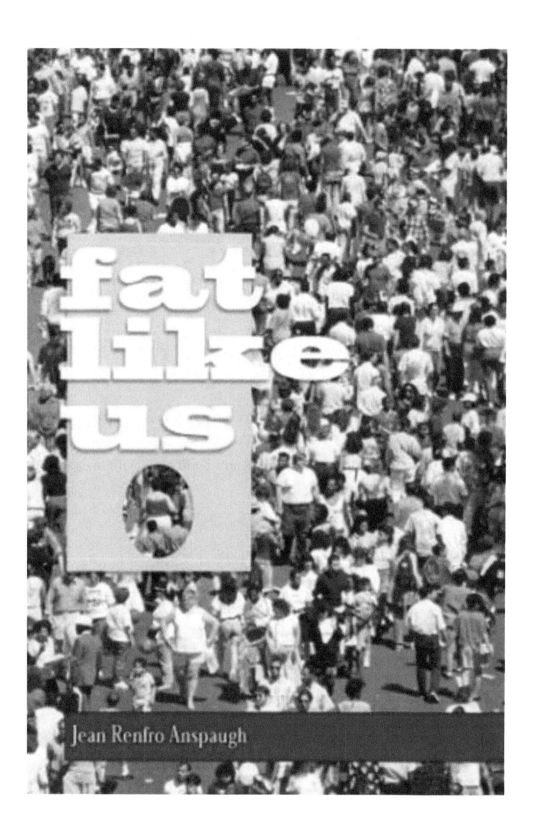

Fig 5-8: Fat like us by Jean Anspaugh is a fun book about what it was like to be a patient of Dr Walter Kempner. Lots of funny lingo in this book about fat people.

According to Jean Anspaugh, "Ricers" had developed their own vocabulary about Durham.

Kempner was the "wizard of Oz," and they were going to the Emerald City.

Alternatively, Kempner was the "**prophet.**" Durham was "**promised land**." Anspaugh says a **fat person wears a "scarlet letter," an "F" for fat everywhere they go**; And after failing all the common diets, they know that they must go to Durham to "**pay for their sins**" and **be redeemed**.

Fat people felt a "**call**," to make a "**pilgrimage**" to Durham.

Dieters knew Durham meant **mild starvation** on a diet of rice & fruits. Last meal before going to Durham was the "**Last Supper**."

Hilton hotel held a dance party for the ricers called "**Crisco Disco**."

A "**chubby chaser**" is a man who dates fat women. "**Whale Watch**" is the pool frequented by ricers.

Jean says, "Fat person is a **caterpillar**, who wants to emerge from their cocoon, like a **butterfly**."

"**Fat like us**" is funny. Entertaining vocabulary & stories. Excellent psychology, and insight into minds of fat people.

Not much nutritional wisdom. Ricers lose weight under guidance of medical staff. Ricers don't seem to learn much about nutrition. Peer pressure culture of rice house helps them to follow the diet & lose weight.

However, when return to their homes & families, they often gain the weight back. Many return to Durham periodically, and some move there.

Jean says "**Hell**" is peak fatness. "**Purgatory**" is loss of motivation, before reaching your weight goal. **Confession** is public weigh ins, and posting ob BP results. Rice & fruit is "**manna**" from Heaven. Rice House is the Temple or Church for dieters.

Morning weigh ins at Rice House were a ricer's religious ritual.

"**Redemption**" or "**renaissance**" was to reach one's weight goal, the "Holy Grail" of dieting. Reset button on one's life.

Routine Kempner have 150-250 pt's in Durham. Kempner waived his fees for poor people.

Pt's lived in hotels, apartments, rooming houses, trailer parks.

Seven days a week: Daily weigh ins, in public, with BP checks were posted on a board for everyone to see, review of blood & urine labs; created peer pressure to follow the diet. Kempner would ask pt's directly, "Did you lose?"

Successful dieters were high status in the group. They were photographed, and their photos passed around to inspire the other dieters.

Someone really ought to make a movie about Kempner & the rice diet.

Dr McDougall newsletter, April 2007, Salt restriction may be good for the heart.

People who lowered their sodium intake by about 2-2.6 grams per day had about a 25% reduction in strokes and heart attacks, even though their blood pressures were reduced by little (-1.7/-.8 mm Hg), or not at all by the salt reduction.

Food companies usually put salt in their foods, because they know that "no salt usually means no sale."

Mentor #3. Roy Swank MD, Phd (1909-2008), was a neurologist from Canada, who later worked in Oregon.

Dr Swank has the best results of any doctor for the treatment of multiple sclerosis (MS) = a 95% reduction in recurrent neurologic events (that's a lot!). Dr McDougall's you tube channel has several videos of Dr Swank. The Swank diet for MS emphasized avoiding saturated fat. Swank diet sets no limits on starches, vegetables, and fruits.

Dr Swank looked at data from Norway. He saw that in dairy areas, eg. central in the country, the incidence of MS was 8x higher. In coastal areas, with little dairy intake, the incidence of MS was low. The distance from the equator was about the same for these areas, so it was NOT a question of the amount of sun exposure available.

Dr Swank also noticed that high fat diets, especially high animal fat, were associated with increased rates of MS. Populations with very low fat diets like China, appeared to have no MS.In WW2, when patients underwent food rationing, and there was less MS.

Dr Swank also studied blood flow. He noticed that high fat meals caused red blood cells to stick together; and this caused hypoxia (decreased oxygen delivery) to adjacent tissues. Dr Swank believes that blood sludge causes tissue hypoxia, and also injures the blood brain barrier.

He then started putting MS patients on low fat diets, and this led to much improved outcomes. The MS patients eating a low fat Swank diet had reduced risk of recurrent MS symptoms, and had a lower risk of heart disease.

Drug therapies for multiple sclerosis, are very expensive, and do not work well. Even with the use of the most modern medications, costing $70,000 a year, the future prospect is dismal, with half of those people afflicted with MS, unable to walk unassisted, bedridden, wheelchair bound, or dead within 10 years of diagnosis.

Roy Swank found that as little as 8 grams per day of saturated fat intake resulted in a threefold increased chance of dying from multiple sclerosis. Saturated fat is very bad for multiple sclerosis patients. **Reference:** Lancet, 1990, Jul 7;336(8706): 37-9.

Reference: Arch neurol 1999 Sep; 56(9):1138-42.

Reference: Mult scler, 2001, Feb; 7(1):59-65.

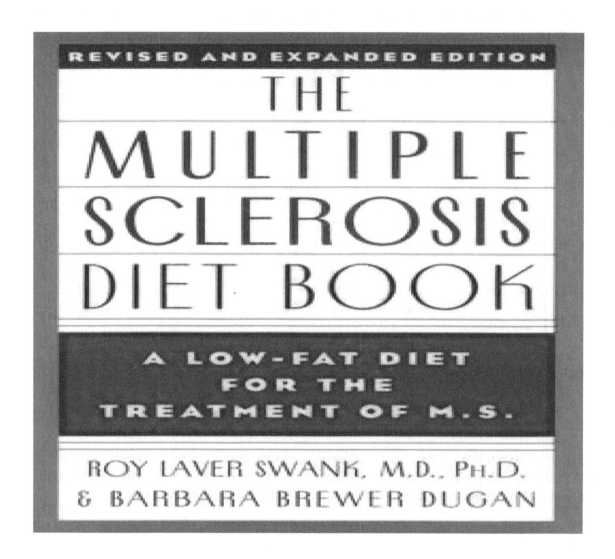

Fig 5-9: Dr Swank's book for treatment of MS.

Roy Swank published a 34 year followup study of his MS patients. Of those who survived the 35 years (ie. did not die of non-MS related diseases) they still were intact for activities of daily living (ADL's) in 95% of the patients. That's an extraordinarily high number of patients.

> Nutrition. 1991 Sep-Oct;7(5):368-76.

Multiple sclerosis: fat-oil relationship

R L Swank [1]

Affiliations + expand
PMID: 1804476

150pt X 34yrs

Abstract

Between 1949 and 1984, 150 patients with multiple sclerosis consumed low-fat diets. Fat, oil, and protein intakes; disability; and deaths were determined. With a daily fat consumption less than 20.1 g/day (av 17 g/day), 31% died, and average deterioration was slight. A daily intake greater than 20 g/day (av 25 or 41 g/day) was attended by serious disability and the deaths of 79 and 81%, respectively. Oil intake bore an indirect relationship to fat consumption. Minimally disabled patients who followed diet recommendations deteriorated little if at all, and only 5% failed to survive the 34 yr of the study, whereas 80% who failed to follow diet recommendations did not survive the study period. The moderately disabled and severely disabled patients who followed diet recommendations carefully did far better than those who failed to follow the diet. In general, women tended to do better than men. Those patients treated early did better than those in whom treatment was delayed. High sensitivity to fats suggests that saturated animal fats are directly involved in the genesis of multiple sclerosis.

Fig 5-10: Saturated fat was especially associated with increased risk of MS.

> Lancet. 1990 Jul 7;336(8706):37-9. doi: 10.1016/0140-6736(90)91533-g.

Effect of low saturated fat diet in early and late cases of multiple sclerosis

R L Swank [1], B B Dugan

Affiliations + expand
PMID: 1973220   DOI: 10.1016/0140-6736(90)91533-g

Abstract

144 multiple sclerosis patients took a low-fat diet for 34 years. For each of three categories of neurological disability (minimum, moderate, severe) patients who adhered to the prescribed diet (less than or equal to 20 g fat/day) showed significantly less deterioration and much lower death rates than did those who consumed more fat than prescribed (greater than 20 g fat/day). The greatest benefit was seen in those with minimum disability at the start of the trial; in this group, when those who died from non-MS diseases were excluded from the analysis, 95% survived and remained physically active.

Fig 5-11: Roy Swank paper. MS patients on a low sat fat diet had much better outcomes on 34 year followup.

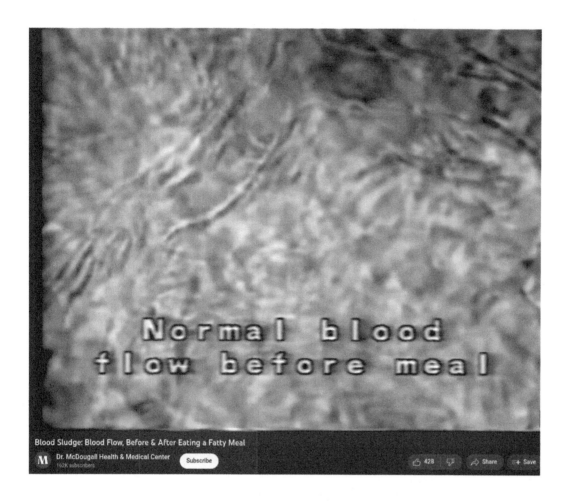

Fig 5-12: This is a great video from Dr McDougall's you tube channel. It's called "Blood sludge: Blood flow, before & after eating a fatty meal. It's only about 50 seconds long. The video was made by Roy Swank.

These types of videos have been made in animals, like hamster cheek pouches, as well as in humans in the eyes, and in the sublingual region.

Before the fatty meal, the RBC zeta potential is intact, and the RBC's are flowing independently of each other.

After the high fat meal, the RBC's became clumped together by the chylomicrons, and this is called blood sludge or rouleaux (stack of coins in French).

The blood sludge also causes decreases oxygen delivery to the tissues. Peter Kuo had measured a 15% drop in oxygen delivery to the tissues.

Roy Swank in hamster brains was able to measure a 30% drop in oxygen delivery to the brain tissue, following a high saturated fat meal.

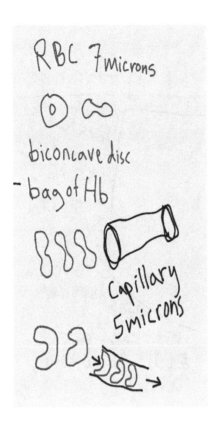

Fig 5-13: Red blood cells are about 7 microns in diameter, and capillaries are about 5 microns in diameter. So RBC's must deform themselves to pass through the capillaries.

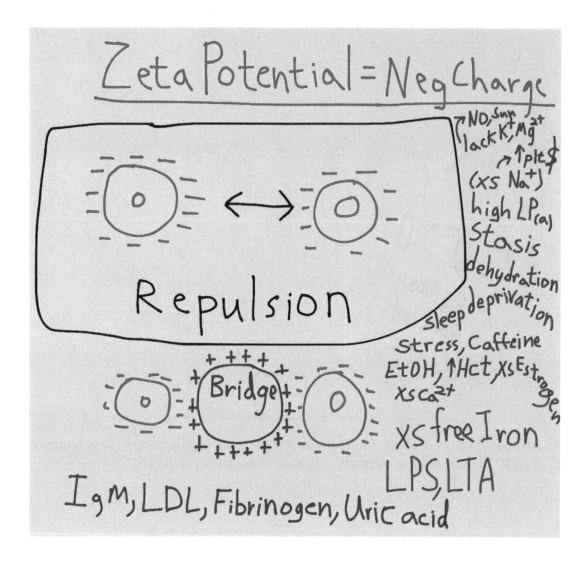

Fig 5-14: Red blood cells have a zeta potential. Zeta potential is the negative charge on their outer surface. The zeta potential arises from the negative charges of cholesterol sulfates, heparan sulfates & sialic acids. When both RBC's have a zeta potential, they repel each other. This is good, because it prevents the RBC's from sticking together.

Bridging molecules overcome the zeta potential and stick RBC's together.

Typical bridging molecules include IgM antibodies, fibrinogen clotting protein, uric acid.

Additional bridging molecules and/or pro-coagulant molecules include: excess boluses of dietary calcium (supplements with daily total above 1,200 mg), excess free iron, excess dietary sodium, excess stress, sleep deprivation, caffeine, dehydration, stasis (sedentary), high LP(a) which is called LP little a, lack of potassium, magnesium, nitrates (nitric oxide precursors), sunshine (increases systemic nitric oxide), excess estrogens.

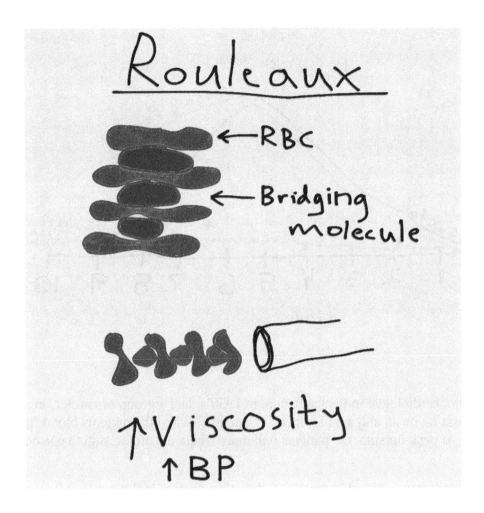

Fig 5-15: Bridging molecules like chylomicrons, LDL cholesterol, uric acid, fibrinogen clotting protein, overcome the zeta potential, and cause RBC's to stick together. When the RBC's are stuck together the blood becomes thicker. Thicker blood is also called increased blood viscosity.

The purpose of blood pressure is to pump blood, against gravity, to the top of your brain. If the blood is thick, the pressure has to go up. It takes higher blood pressure to pump thick blood (like a milkshake) to the top of your brain, than to pump normal blood (like water).

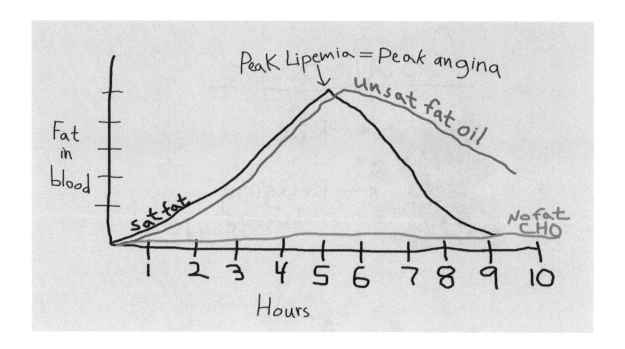

Fig 5-16: Peter Kuo, cardiologist in Pennsylvania, in 1950's, had a group of cardiac angina patients eat a high sat fat meal, and a no fat meal. Then he checked the patients blood lipids every 30 minutes. At peak lipemia, the patients had more frequent cardiac angina episodes.[3]

These types of studies were repeated in the 1960's by other doctors including Ray Rosenman & Meyer Friedman.[4] They showed that omega 6 cooking oils caused an even more prolonged sludging of the blood. The work of Meyer Friedman, Ray Rosenman, Roy Swank, and Peter Kuo showed that one high fat meal can reduce the arterial pressure of oxygen (PaO2) by 20%.

Reference: see footnotes on this page for papers by Kuo and Friedman.

Note that the blood did not sludge after the carbohydrate meal with no fat, and these patients did not have anginal episodes.

3Kuo (1955) "**Angina pectoris induced by fat ingestion** in patients with coronary artery disease" JAMA 158: 1008-13.

4 Friedman (1965) "**Effect of unsaturated fats upon lipemia & conjunctival circulation**" JAMA 193: 882-86

Mentor #4. Nathan Pritikin.

f you want to study English literature, you should first learn about Greek mythology, and the Bible. If you want to study Nutrition literature, you should first learn about Kempner, Pritikin, and McDougall.

Nathan Pritikin, at 40 years of age, was diagnosed with moderate to severe coronary artery disease, based on treadmill stress test, and abnormal EKG. His total chol 300.

He then studied nutrition and atherosclerosis with the hope of saving his own life. He became a vegetarian, and started exercising

He figured out how to cure himself in 11 years. At his repeat treadmill stress test he ran for 20 minutes with no trace of coronary ischemia.

Chiron the centaur was wounded by an arrow. Chiron searched for knowledge to heal himself. While learning to help himself, he learned how to help others.

"The doctor is effective only when he himself is affected. Only the wounded   physician heals. The pains and burdens one bears, and eventually overcomes, are the source of great wisdom, and healing power for others."   - Carl Jung (1875-1961).

He noticed that the USA or Western diet was high fat, high sugar, and low fiber. He noticed that the countries that eat high fat diets have high rates of degenerative diseases like obesity, hypertension, diabetes, coronary artery disease, impotence, osteoarthritis, autoimmune disease, hearing loss, and vidion loss.

Hearing loss due to atherosclerosis and ischemia is much more common in Western countries.

Pritikin noticed that when Walter Kempner put his patients on low fat diet, the results were good. Pritikin noticed that populations eating low fat, plant based diets, like the Tarahumara in Northern Mexico had incredible endurance.

Tarahumara can run 100 miles in three days, carrying a heavy pack. The Tarahumara diet is 80:10:10, carbohydrate, protein, fat.

In comparison, the Pima population in Arizona, who are genetically similar to the Tarahumara, eat the SAD diet, and have lots of obesity, hypertension, diabetes, coronary artery disease, and gallstones.

93

Pritikin also noticed that populations eating high fat diets have high rates of cancer.

Pritikin concluded that excess dietary fat was the main cause of chronic disease. Pritikin said that diets are best categorized based on the amount of fat they contain.

Pritikin used the word "LipoToxemia" to describe the pattern of high fat diets causing many chronic diseases.

Pritikin said that high fat diets were especiall bad for 3 reasons: #1. tissue hypoxia. #2. diabetes. #3. elevated cholesterol, and this leading to increased atheroslcerosis.

Pritikin famously said, **"Fat is bad."**

Pritikin also famously said, "There's no such thing as a [naturally occuring] fat deficient diet."

Pritikin searched the scientific literature on dietary fat, and found that a patient cohort was fed .75% of calories from fat (less than 1%) and did very well.

Pritikin started out recommending to keep dietary fat as a percentage of calories, as below 15%; but gradually moved towards recommending to keep fat below 105 of calories.

Pritikin did allow a minimal amout of animal food for obtaining vitamin B12, and for patient acceptance.

Drs Esselstyn, McDougall, T. Colin Campbell, Peter Rogers recommend zero% of calories from animal foods. Vitamin B12 can be obtained by taking methyl cobalamin pills.

In some videos Dr McDougall recommended against taking cyanocobalamin. In another video, he said it was okay to take cyanocobalamin, and that he has taken all three types of B12 = methyl-cobalamin, hydroxy-cobalamin & cyano-cobalamin.

[I only take methyl-cobalamin, and would never take cyano-cobalamin].

Nathan Pritikin and John McDougall MD especially emphasize the role of high fat diets in causing obesity, hypertension, diabetes, and atherosclerosis.

Walter Kempner MD and Richard Moore MD, Phd especially emphasized the role of excess dietary sodium, (and the relative lack of potassium & magnesium) to causing hypertension.

Dr McDougall's you tube channel has a video interview with Nathan Pritikin.

Reference: **Dr McDougall newsletter, February 2013, Nathan Pritikin – McDougall's most important mentor. (includes video interview with Pritikin, 1982).**

The you tube channel TB1M1 has 6.2 video hours of Nathan Pritikin lectures.

Programs ⌄ **Dr.McDougall®** Shop

sing. A visionary physician and author, beloved husband, father, grandfather, brother, mentor and friend, Dr. McDougall died p

Nathan Pritikin: A Review of Medical Literature on Relationships of Various Degenerative Diseases to Diet and Activity

The fundamentals of the McDougall Program are simple yet often difficult to implement. Learn about the *12-Day McDougall Program* - a life-saving medical program that empowers participants with the knowledge and practical steps needed to live a vibrant, long life. For questions on whether a change in diet can help your ailment, learn more about our *consultations*.

Learn more

Nathan Pritikin was the scientific pioneer who thirty years ago told people the cause and cure of our common chronic diseases. His work is presented in scientific detail in the attached review of the medical literature.

A Review of the Medical Literature

Also See:

The McDougall February 2013 newsletter more on Mr. Pritikin and a video interview

Fig 5-17: Nathan Pritikin's legacy book is available free at the Dr McDougall dot com website.

Chapter 6. **Starch Solution**

"Starch has unlocked the door to good health for thousands of my patients" – Dr John McDougall.

Dr McDougall did his internal medicine internship in Hawaii. After internship, he worked in Hawaii, taking care of patients from a sugar plantation, and from an city population.

He noticed that the sugar plantation workers tended to remain slim, active, and free of medications into their nineties.

He noticed that the people eating starch based diets were had no diabetes or coronary artery disease, and very little breast cancer, prostate cancer or colon cancer.

He noticed that with Asian populations, (Chinese, Japanese, Korean, Philipines) emigrating to the USA, the grandparents were usually thin and healthy; their children heavier, and not as healthy; the grandchildren were the heaviest and the sickest, because of the SAD (Standard American Diet) diet.

Dr McDougall recalled that nutrition had almost never been mentioned in medical school, medical textbooks or residency.

Yet, it was this experience in Hawaii that provided the most valuable insight.

When people adopted a plant based, starch based diet, they were routinely able to improve their bodyweight, to be able to come off many pills, and were less likely to need surgeries.

"I went to the Hawaii medical library, and saw study after study that described weight loss, relief of chest pain, headaches, arthritis, owing to a simple solution:

a diet based on starch, supplemented by vegetables and fruits.

No pills or surgery needed…

Healthy populations get most of their calories from starch.

In fact, all long term healthy populations get most of their calories from starch.

There are no exceptions.

The same truth dates back through recorded human history.

Asians ate **rice**. Okinawans also ate **sweet potatos.**

The Mayans and Aztecs were known as people of the **corn.**

The Incas of South America ate **potatos and quinoa.**

The ancient Egyptians ate **Wheat**." - Dr McDougall.

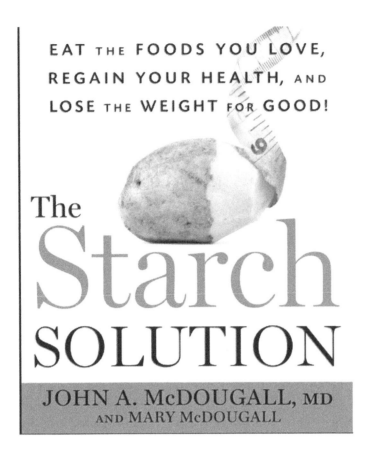

Fig 6-1: Starch Solution by John McDougall MD is one of the best nutrition, health, medical books ever written.

Starch is what you do!

Epidemiology is how you know it's true!

If a person eats a starch based, whole food, vegan diet, then they almost certainly will be thin with no type 2 diabetes, and a good blood pressure, and clean coronary arteries, and a relatively low risk of cancer.

Dr McDougall figured this out.

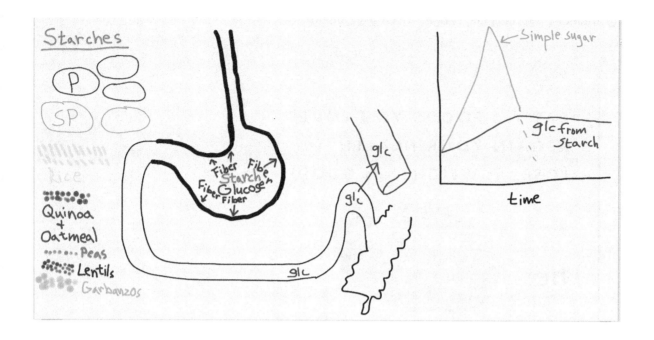

Fig 6-2: Starch is low caloric density, so it stretches the stomach with relatively few calories; Stretching the stomach provides early satisfaction of hunger.

Then the starch goes into the small bowel. Starch is a polymer (means bunch of connected molecules) of glucose wrapped in fiber.

The small bowel enzymes need time to separate the glucose from the fiber. This gives starch the "effect" of being like a slow, gradual release energy "pill."

Glucose is slowly absorbed from the gut to the blood. This keeps the blood glucose level in a good range for a prolonged amount of time. This satisfies hunger for a prolonged amount of time.

This satisfies hunger with the fewest calories, so starch eating populations are thin.

"Starch is the best food to satisfy hunger" – Dr John McDougall.

"Starch should be our primary source of digestible carbohydrate... digestion of starches is a slow process that gradually releases the sugars from starch; which then goes from the intestine to the blood.

fruits offer a quick burning energy, mostly in the form of simple sugars, but little of slow burning, sustaining starch.

As a result, fruits alone won't satisfy our appetites for very long...

We humans are built to thrive on starch. The more starch we consume, the healthier we become.

Starches include rice, corn, potatoes, sweet potatoes, beans, peas, barley, millet, oats, rye, sorghum, wheat, squash.-

"If you take just one message from this book, it should be: **EAT MORE STARCH.**" Humans are **STARCHIVORES**." – Dr John McDougall.

If a person eats simple sugars, like soda pop, there is a tendency to rapidly spike up the blood glucose level, and then for the pancreas to overcompensate, releasing a large amount of insulin; this rapidly drives down the blood glucose level, and can lead to rebound hypoglycemia.

"75% of disease in industrialized countries is **chronic dietary problems** like obesity, HTN, cad, dm, arthritis, cancer...

What do these people have in common?

A diet dominated by meat, dairy, fat & processed foods

For a dz to progress → injury must OUTPACE healing.

For healing to occur → healing must outpace ongoing injury.

If injury goes on too long → will eventually do irreversible damage.

The body is always trying to heal. It does not stop; not even for 1 second.

During my early years in Hawaii, a young man mangled by a **motorcycle accident,** had many broken ribs, a skull fracture, a left thigh comminuted open fracture, and numerous superficial lacerations.

Within a week, he was walking with crutches

After 3 months, he was walking on his own without a limp

If a body can heal from this massive assault, then it can heal from almost anything" – Dr John McDougall.

"If we eat natural plant foods, we will **ALWAYS , DURING ALL STAGES OF LIFE, GET ENOUGH DHA, AND OTHER OMEGA 3 FATS.** - Dr John McDougall, from Starch Solution, p. 123

Fish don't make omega 3 fats. The fish gets the omega 3 fats from the plants. It's the algae and

101

the seaweed that makes the omega 3's.

A fat is a fat is a fat....

Serial angiograms of human heart arteries over a year of study showed that all three types of fat – sat fat (animal fat), MUFA (olive oil), PUFA (O3&6 oils) –

were all associated with significant increases in new atherosclerotic lesions.

Decreasing total fat intake was the ONLY way to stop the [atherosclerosis] lesions from growing...

One of the most important predictors of hear attack risk is an elevated level of factor 7, a substance that enables blood clotting.

Reference: Larsen et al. Effects of dietary fat quality and quantity on postprandial activation of blood coagulation factor 7, arterioscler thromb vasc biol, 1997, Nov; 17(11):2904-9.

Formation of clots inside of the arteries causes most heart attacks and strokes.

Olive oil increases blood clottting activity by increasing clostting factor 7 as much as animal fats do.

Vegetable oils also impair circulation resulting in a 20% reduction in blood oxygen.

Reduced oxygen circulation can lead to angina (chest pain), impaired brain function, and fatigue." Dr John McDougall from Starch Solution, pp. 135-136

Ref: Kuo, P. The effect of lipemia upon coronary and peripheral arterial circulation in patiatients with essential hyperlipemia. Am J Med 1959, Jan; 26(1):68-75.

"Nuts and seeds have about 805 of calories from fat... Soy has about 40% of calories from fat... grains and legumes have about 5-10% of calories from fat." - Dr McDougall, from Starch Solution p. 137.

Soy has some estrogenic effects. Soy can change a women's menstrual cycle.

Endometrial ablation by heating or by cooling is a procedure that stops menstruation.

"Soy protein increases ILGF more than does cow protein. Soy isolated protein increases ILGF-1 (insulin like growth factor – 1) almost twice as much as cow milk protein: milk concentrate 36% incease ILGF vs soy concentrate with 69% increase ILGF. **Reference:** j clin endocrinol metab, 2003, Mar, 88(3): 1048-54. The concern is that something that increases ILGF-1 might increase cancer risk.

"It's okay to eat small amounts of minimally processed soy, like 2 oz or less, but it's not a health food." - Dr John McDougall from video **Dr McDougall disputes major medical treatments – osteroporosis, and the broken bone business.**

"Fat is the real culprit in weight gain and causing illness… Salt and sugar are the scapegoats of the Western diet…

The eskimo diet is 50% fat, 35% protein & 15% carbohydrate.

the western diet is 40% fat, 20% protein & 40% carbohydrate.

The McDougall diet is 8% fat, 12% protein & 80% carbohydrate…

The Kempner diet is 5% fat, 5% protein & 90% carbohydrate…

Reference: Dr McDougall newsletter, April 2015, extreme nutrition, the diet of eskimos.

you gotta let people put a little salt and sugar on their plant foods, or most won't eat them… dietary sugar does not cause type 2 diabetes… " - Dr John McDougall.

Dr McDougall does say that an excess consumption of simple sugars can lead to elevated blood triglycerides, which is associated with increased risk of heart attack and stroke. - Starch Solution , p. 183.

"A muscle is a muscle is a muscle… Because many fish are high on the food chain, they are highly contaminated with enviromental chemicals… high content of mercury… fish is high in fat – often 60% of the calories come from fat… contributing to obesity…

there is considerable evidence that fish fat (omega 3) will increase a person's risk of cancer, and also will increase the risk of metastasis…

fish fat is known to paralyze the actions of insulin, and increase the tendency for diabetes, and to suppress the immune system… even when fish oil is purified of cholesterol, the omega 3 fat itself will cause the LDL-bad cholesterol to rise… fish oil treatment does NOT promote favorable changes in the diameter of atherosclerotic coronary arteries..." - Dr McDougall, newsletter, February 2003.

Chapter 7. **Gastrointestinal tuneup**

Gastrointestinal tuneup by Dr John McDougall is another great book.

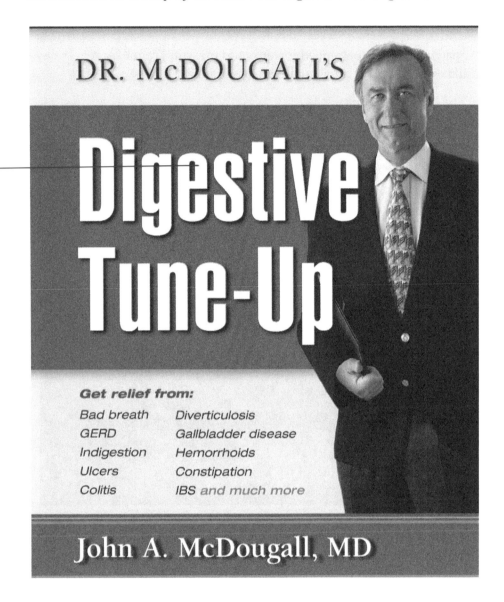

Fig 7-1: Gastrointestinal tuneup by John McDougall.

"Prevention is always the preferred option...

I'm the luckiest Dr in the world, b/c my pt's regain their lost health & appearance by

Following the simple, cost free, side effect free, dietary & lifestyle advice I prescribe...

The food you put into your body is the SINGLE MOST POWERFUL FACTOR THAT DETERMINES YOUR HEALTH & WELL BEING...

105

I will tell you my story how I was transformed from a chronically ill young man to a person who could be considered **the picture of health at 59 years** of age (born in 1947).

I regularly windsurf in the deep blue ocean, and strap my grandson into a backpack, and carry him on a mountain hiking adventure. P xi

Through dietary change… patients have experienced lower blood pressure, relief from headaches, arthritis pain, and even in many cases, complete healing of dz's like

Type 2 dm, obesity, RA, Ht dz (actually reversing atherosclerosis) without medication" – John McDougall MD from Gastrointestinal tuneup.

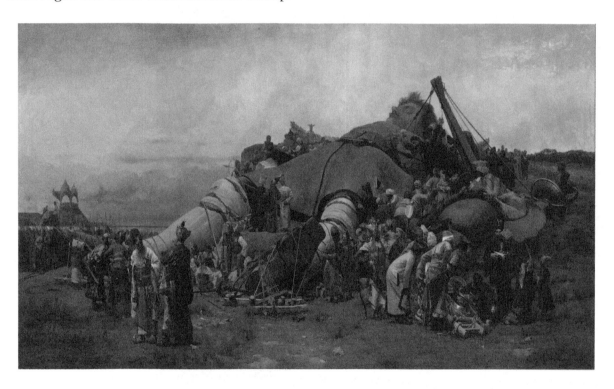

Fig 7-2: Gulliver & Lilliputians by Jehan Georges Vibert, 1900, public domain. The difference in healing ability for the chronic western diseases, of a doctor who knows nutirition & epidemiology vs a regular doctor, is like the difference between a Gulliver & Lilliputians.

Food is the major determining factor in how we **smell** to others.

Bad breath is especially due to eating animal foods, because they have more sulfur containing amino acids, like methionine and cysteine... **if you eat it, you ooze it!** - Dr John McDougall from Gastrointestinal tuneup.

"Dairy (especially the dairy protein = so this occurs with low fat dairy and skim milk) paralyzes the bowel muscles, and leads to constipation… High fat diet are associated with increased heartburn. Excess dietary fat can cause heartburn = peaks 3 hr after a high fat meal.

Other causes of constipation include #1. a low fiber diet. #2. Calcium channel blockers. #3. excess stress.

Eating more plant foods, which provides more dietary fiber, helps to prevent constipation. When making the diet change from SAD diet to a plant based diet, one can drink some prune juice to help alleviate constipation.

If a person should need a laxative, then lactulose is the best one. Mineral oil is okay for treatment of constipation.

Coffee (including decaf) increases risk of LES (Lower Esophagel Sphincter) dysfunction & GERD (GastroEsophageal Reflux Disease). Cigarettes & EtOH cause LES dysfunction & GERD.

Over 90% of gallstones (GS) are cholesterol gallstones… The higher the amount of animal foods, the higher the amount of GS.

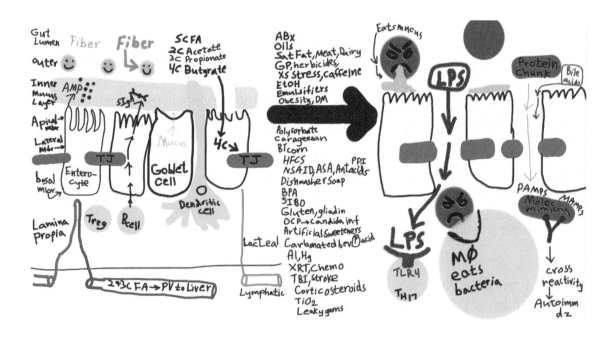

Fig 7-3: The intestinal barrier = gut wall = gut epithelium = enterocytes. The gut is called the enteric tract. Cytes means cells. Enterocytes = gut lining cells. Gut wall is one cell thick. That's it. In between enterocytes, there are tight junctions.

The good gut bacteria convert dietary fiber into short chain fatty acids. Butyrate is the most important of the short chain fatty acids. Enterocytes use the butyrate to make tight junctions.

Lack of dietary fiber tends to lead to leaky gut. Leaky gut is also called "inreased intestinal permeability. Leaky gut greatly increases the risk inflammatory bowel disease, and of autoimmune disease.

107

"Mild chronic colits is most often referred to as IBS (irritable bowel syndrome) = abnormal bowel function, with episodes of both diarrhea & constipation. IBS is the most common cause of referral to gastroenterologist = about 50% of visits.

The most common cause of IBS is milk (lactose), wheat, eggs, and high fat diet. For IBS, the McDougall diet is usually a good treatment" – Dr McDougall from Gastrointestinal tuneup, p. 96.

"Inflammatory Bowel dieases include ulcerative colitis and Crohn's disease. IBD is found exclusively in persons eating a western diet.

IBD is more common in northern populations, because they eat more meat and dairy. Crohn's dz pts can have > 20 stools per day. The tend to find relief from watery stools with the McDougall diet within 3 days. Pt's with UC & Crohns greatly benefit from a low fat plant based diet

"The best way to prevent and treat all forms of colitis from mild to severe is to ELIMINATE ALL FREE FATS (VEGETABLE OILS) & ANIMAL PRODUCTS

and to begin consuming a starch based diet withfruits and vegetables. if that doesn't work, then eliminate all wheat products" - Dr McDougall from Gastrointestinal tuneup p. 102.

"Offending foods for celiac dz = barley, kamut, rye, spelt, triticale, wheat (semolina, durum, bulgur, seitan), beer, ales, malted drinks.

Foods acceptable for celiac dz = rice, millet, some oats, buckwheat (kasha), corn, quinoa, potatos, sweet potatos, legumes, green & yellow veggies, all fruits" – Dr McDougall from Gastrointestinal tuneup, p. 99.

"Colon Polyps are a cellular proliferation of mucus membrane, in response to constant irritation.

"Irritation leads to cell proliferation; cell proliferation leads to small polyp development. Small polyps grow into larger polyp. With large polyps, some cells sometimes turn into cancer.

Larger the polyp the farther along it is towards becoming cancer. Colon cancer risk is strongly linked to diet. SAD diet = high risk for colon cancer. Low fat PBD = low risk for colon cancer.

Animal fat, cholesterol, and animal protein all increase risk of colon polyps & colon cancer risk.

Sulfur amino acids lead to increased Hydrogen Sulfite in colon which is toxic to gut wall

Increased dietary fat leads to increased bile acids in colon. Lack of fiber leads to bad gut bacteria that produce chemicals toxic to gut wall. Fiber is converted by good gut bacteria into butyrate and this inhibits the growth of colon cancer cells.

Just increasing our fiber intake by 13 g/d is thought to reduce risk of colon cancer by 31%.

There is substantial evidence that a low fat no cholesterol diet can slow the growth of colon cancer, and allow a person a longer, healthier life.

Stop eating animal foods & oils! = stop throwing gasoline on the fire!" - Dr McDougall, pp. 110-114.

"Fat, female, fair, fertile, flatulent, forty are all associated with increased risk of having gallstones in the gallbladder. About 30% of Americans over 60 years of age have gallstones. About 1% of them have serious symptoms.

Gallstones are usually cholesterol gallstones, at least 90% of them. The bile becomes super saturated from cholesterol, and it precipitates to form cholesterol gallstones. Cholesterol only comes from animal foods.

When the gallbladder is surgically removed (cholecystectomy), the bile has nowhere to be stored. **The bile, slowly, continuously drips into the small bowel. This can lead to irritation of the colon, and diarrhea. This leads to increased risk of right sided colon cancer**….

If you have asymptomatic gallstones, it is best to leave them alone, and to just eat the McDougall diet.

What do you think causes the liver to be infiltrated by fat? The same thing that causes fat accumulation everywhere else. Eating fat!

This idea of "good fats" is toxic! Don't buy into the this "good fats" stuff. So called "good fats" increase your risk of obesity and cancer.

LOW FAT is the way you want to go.

For patients with liver disease, a low protein diet is easier on the liver. Plant proteins are easier on the liver.

Subcutaneous lipomas sometimes decrease when a patient loses weight…

Cellulite disappears with weight loss…

Acne does not occur in teenagers where people eat low fat diets.

- From How to prevent fatty liver From Dr M YT channel.

Dr McDougall newsletter, Feb 2002. My stomach's on fire, and I can't put it out.

Detailed discussion of GERD, and related conditions, symptoms and treatment.

Chapter 8. **Obesity & fat**

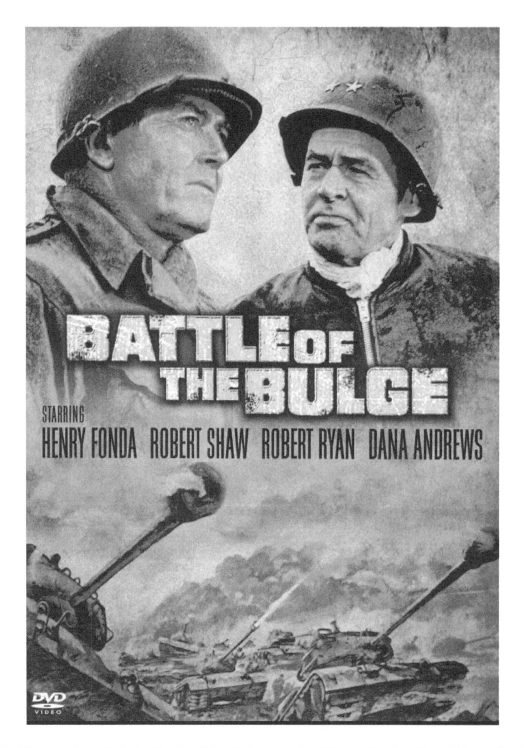

Fig 8-1: The movie called the Battle of the Bulge starring Henry Fonda. Dr McDougall said the struggle to control one's body weight was the **"Battle of the Bulge."**

Dr McDougall newsletter, Feb 2006, moderation is impossible for passionate people.

Have you ever seen a smoker quit by "cutting down?" I haven't. Have you ever hear of an alcoholic who sobered up by "switching to beer?" I haven't.

The only effective means to overcome these destructive habits is to remove the powerful substance from the person's life.

Extreme change returns tremendous rewards. Eating the low fat vegan diet, a person loses weight faster; and it's sustainable.

Throughout my entire life, I have been enthusiastic about everything… I was born this way. So now, even if I wanted to, I could not become a "moderate" person. So I have found the solution.

I now direct my energies towards supportive, not destructive, behaviors. I have learned to love healthy foods.

Irish poet and dramatist Oscar Wilde said, "Moderation is a fatal thing. Nothing succeeds like excess."

Dr McDougall newsletter November & December 2015, Food, sex, and attractiveness.

Health is attractive. Men and women want to mate with the healthiest person possible. Good health suggests the parents will be better able to provide a safe shelter and adequate food. Good health predicts longevity.

Testosterone is 13% higher in male vegans, than in meat eaters. Men who consume meat and dairy are likely to become impotent earlier in life.

Low fat diets lead to better blood flow, to better tissue oxygenation, and this gives the skin a glow of vitality that is attractive.

Low fat, vegan diets reduce the risk of acne.

Animal protein has more sulfur containing amino acids like methionine and cysteine. These lead to bad breath which is called halitosis. This also causes smelly farts.

For this chapter, I watched the videos about obesity and dietary fat at the Dr McDougall (Dr M) Health & Medical Center you tube (YT) channel. **Video titles are in blue ink.**

"The fat you eat is the fat you wear… it goes from the lips to the hips… the primary purpose of fat is for storage; for the day when you have no food… it moves so effortlessly from your gut to your body, that **I can tell what type of fat you eat with a biopsy needle**. I can biopsy your buttocks, and the type of fat will match what you eat…

113

Saturated fat and cholesterol are euphemisms for animal foods. Complex carbohydrate is a euphemism for starch. Starch is the Germanic root word with the meanings of strong, stiff, strengthen, stiffen. By describing foods in these ways, the problems with animal foods are hidden; and the benefits of starch are hidden.

It is much better to call starch foods what they are, which is starches, than to call them complex carbohydrates. People know what starches are; at least my grandmother knew what starches were. When we were going to visit grandma, she would say, "What starch will you be having?"

Almost no one knows what a complex carbohydrate is. How would an average person respond if you asked them what complex carbohydrates do you like?

Omega 3 fats increase the risk of bleeding… the **omega 3 fats also suppress the immune system**… they make you less able to fight an infection or cancer… **omega 6 fats in oils are even more toxic to the arteries than is saturated fat**…

The two essential fats, omega 3 and omega 6, are both, only made by plants. Fish do not make omega 3 fats. Fis get them from eating algae and seaweed.

All free oils are highly processed foods, and should be considered drugs, not foods; all drugs have adverse side effects… oil is 9 calories per gram, which is the highest possible amount of calories… Starch is only 1 calorie per gram…

Free oils are added to processed foods to get stuff to stick to them. Eg. oil on french fries gets the salt to stick to them. Oil on a donut gets the sugar to stick to it. These free oils are toxic, and cause increased risk of cancer.

natural plant foods do contain small amounts of oil, but they are not free. These small amounts of oil are "packaged" inside the plant in a way that protects them, and you.

a starch based diet has all the fats you need, including for omega 3; and they're in the proper amount, and the proper enviroment; so the fat isn't toxic, like it is when it comes in a bottle.

- John McDougall (Dr M) from video at his YT (you tube) channel, **"Is there such a thing as "healthy fats?" and potato mastermind lecture part 1.**

When friends ask: Why do you avoid adding vegetable oils? August 2007 Newsletter by Dr McDougall.

The main distinction between a "fat" and an "oil" is whether they're solid or liquid at room temperature.

Free oils are drugs. Free oils are NOT food.

Only plants can make omega 3 and omega 6 fats. The essential omega 3 fat is Alpha Linolenic Acid (ALA). The essential omega 6 fat is Linoleic acid (LA). Longer chain omega 3 and omega 6 fatty acids can be built from these. [ALA & LA are the "parent" essential fatty acids that the human body can make into longer fatty acids.]

Our dietary requirements for o3 & o6 fats is very minimal, and can be readily obtained from a plant based diet; so in practical terms, "essential fatty acid deficiency" is essentially unknown in free living populations.

Omega 3 oils suppress the immune system; and have been used as medications for autoimmune diseases; the reports of their benefit are variable, and often questionable.

Eating oils increases the risk of weight gain.

All three types of fat = sat fat (animal fat), monounsaturated (olive oil) and PUFA (polyunsaturated fatty acids) o3 & o6 fats were associated with significant increases in new atherosclerotic lesions over 1 year of study.   Only by decreasing intake of ALL fats did the lesions stop growing. **Reference:** Blankenhorn et al. Influence of diet on the appearance of new lesions in human coronary arteries. Jama, 1990, Mar 23-30;263(12):1646-52.

"Olive oil is toxic for humans. All oils are." - Dr McDougall

In a study of African green monkeys [their physiology is thought similar to humans], when sat fat was replaced with olive oil, there was no protection from atherosclerosis. **Reference:** Rudel et al. Compared with dietary monounsaturated and saturated fat, polyunsaturated fat protects African green monkes from coronary artery atherosclerosis. Arterioscler thromb vasc biol, 1995, Dec; 15(12):2101-10.

All five fats tested, canola oil, olive oil, sunflower oil, palm oil, and butter causes increases in blood triglycerides and clotting factor #7. **Reference:** Larsen LF et al. Effects of dietary fat quality and quantity on postprandial activation of blood coagulation factor 7. Aterioscler thromb vasc biol, 1997, Nov;17(11):2904-9.

Research on animals suggests that o6 oils are very cancer promoting.

In one animal experiment on colon cancer, a fish oil diet induced 10x more metastases, than a low fat diet. **Reference:** Griffini P. Dietary omega 3 fatty acids promote colon carcinoma metastasis in rat liver. Cancer res, 1998, Aug 1:58(15) 3312-9.

Population studies world wide tell us that that the lower the total fat intake, the less the risk of common cancers, such as breast, colon, and prostate. **Reference:** Carroll K, Experimental evidence of dietary factors and hormone dependent cancers. Cancer res, 1975, Nov;35(11 pt 2):3374-83.

Many people say, "I'm vegan, but I'm still overweight." They often are still eating oils. They need to take the final step, and just say no to oils.

Omega 3 supplements worsen type 2 diabetics. Reference. elevated plasma glucose and lowered triglyceride levels from omega 3 fatty acid supplementation in type 2 diabetes. By John Ensinck et al. Diabetes care, 1989, Apr, 12(4):276-81. After omega 3 fatty acid supplementation (8 grams per day for 8 weeks) the fasting plasma glucose levels increased 22%… postprandial blood glucose levels increased 35%. - Dr John McDougall.

Blood sludge: Blood flow, before & after eating a fatty meal (courtesy of Roy Swank MD, animal arteries shown) at Dr M YT channel. ALL HEALTH CARE PROVIDERS SHOULD WATCH THIS VIDEO!! It's only 52 seconds long. It shows how a fatty meal causes the RBC's to stick together = blood sludge.

"Other words for fat people include chubby, portly, stout, heavyset, plump, rotund, buxom, very well rounded…2/3 of population is overweight or obese… **nature is perfect;** it knows how to design animals.

Human obesity is not because people are designed wrong. **It's not because of the genes. It's because they are eating the wrong food**…

It used to be only Kings and Queens could eat all these high fat foods, and they got fat; now most of the industrialized population can, and they are getting fat…

There are only 5 ways to lose weight: #1. You can starve = portion control diet. #2. You can make yourself sick. Eg. with the low carb, keto diet. The ketosis is like starvation, and it dulls the appetite. Ketosis can result in a profound loss of appetite. The keto diet causes weight loss by making the patient sick. It's the the make yourself sick diet.

You lose 6-8 lbs of water weight the first week from the loss of glycogen [it's stored bound to water]. #3. You can have bariatric surgery. #4. You can take diet pills or injections like ozempic (similar to gila monster venom). **#5. You can eat a starch based diet.** This is the best option by far.

There are 3 key things about the **starch based diet that make it the best for weight loss:** 1. It's low caloric density. 2. It's low fat. 3. It has lots of carbohydrates to satisfy hunger.

Inability to satisfy the hunger drive is the main reason why weight loss diets fail. Starch prevents this problem, because starch is the best food to satisfy hunger.

Experiments were done where the amount of fat in the food was hidden from the study subjects: in the form of butter, mayonaise, vegetable oil, margarine that had been added to soups, stews, muffins, breads, sandwiches, deserts.

When the subjects were fed food with the fat largely removed, they unknowingly ate 600 fewer calories. Conclusion: "These results suggest that habitual unrestriced consumption of low fat diets may be an effective approach to weight control.

Reference: Am j clin nutr, 1987, Dec; 46(6):886-92.

Reference: J clin invest, 1985, Sep; 76(3):1019-24.

Reference: Dr McDougall newsletter, April 2004, "Good" HDL cholesterol is meaningless.

Reference: Dr McDougall was fired from speaking at the obesity medicine conference. Dr McDougall newsletter, March 2016

Reference: Dr McDougall newsletter January 2003, taming elevated triglycerides, insulin resistance, and syndrome x.

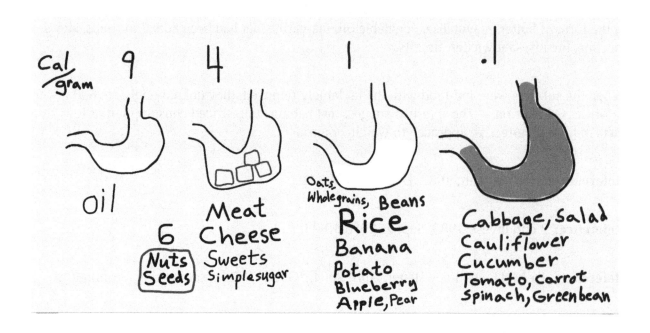

Fig 8-2: Caloric density of different foods. Oil is liquid fat. It takes a lot of calories of oil to stretch the stomach. Stretch of the stomach provides early satisfaction of hunger.

Notice that nuts and seeds are 70-90% fat which means very high caloric density.

Meat, cheese & sweets have high caloric density.

Starch has much lower caloric density; about 1 calorie per gram. Sweet fruits like apples, pears, blueberries has almost as much caloric density as the common starches like rice, beans, oatmeal.

Veggies have very low caloric density. So it's good to eat a lot of veggies when trying to lose weight.

Low caloric density means that relatively few calories will STRETCH the stomach, and this provides early satisfaction of hunger. Then the glucose is gradually absorbed, and this causes longer satisfaction of hunger…

pure white sugar is 4 calories per gram….

Oils, butter, margarine, salad dressings are 100% fat.

Meat and cheese are about 60-70% fat.

White sugar is 0% fat.

Potatos are 1% fat.

The body prefers to store fat, and **to burn carbohydrate.** The brain, the kidney, and the RBC's especially prefer to burn carbohydrate... You can tell what type of fat a person eats by a biopsy of their fat. "Studies of adipose tissue in man" by Stoffel, Am J clin nutr, 1960, 8:499-511…

De novo lipogenesis **(conversion of dietary sugars to fat)** is too metabolically inefficient, such that the body seldom does it; **it's insignificant in humans**...

Just look around. Are rice eaters fat? Are potato eaters fat? It costs 30% of calories to convert glucose into fat. So the body prefers to burn glucose.

It costs only 3% of calories to simply store fat as fat.

High fat foods are NOT good at satisfying hunger. That's why people overeat them; and this leads to excess intake of fat, and this leads to obesity…

Carbohydrates are what satisfies the hunger drive…

Our mouths are different from carnivores. Cats do not have taste buds for sweets or starchy foods. Humans do… Cats have big teeth for piercing flesh. Humans don't. Cats have 7x more stomach acid than humans, because they need it for digesting the high protein meat. Carnivores have a short digestive tract. Humans have a long digestive tract…

The foods that make you fat, also make you sick. **The foods that make you trim, also make you healthy**…

The McDougall Diet

I recommend you eat about 90% of your calories from starches. And the other 10% should be fruits and veggies. That's the McDougall diet…

Papers showing the benefits of the McDougall die include:

Reference: Effects of 7 days on an ad libitum low fat vegan diet: the McDougall program cohort. Nutr j 13, 99, (2014). In 7 days showed an average total cholesterol reduction of 22 mg/dL; and showed blood pressure reduction of -18/11 mm HG.

Reference: Low fat, plant based diet in multiple sclerosis: a randomized controlled trial. Mult scler relat disord, 9, 80, (2016). In twelve months the total cholesterol average was reduced.

119

Reference: The BROAD study: a randomized controlled trial using a whole food plant based diet in the community for obesity, ischaemic heart disease or diabetes." Nutr & diabetes, 7, e256, (2017). Total cholesterol was reduced at twelve months by -20.0 mg/d.

Below ground plant storage foods like potatos and sweet potatos are nutritionally complete, except for vitamin B12.

Above ground plant storage organs like grains (corn, rice, wheat) and legumes (beans, lentils, peas) and seeds are deficient in vitamins A & C... Vitamins A & C are easily obtained by eating a little bit of fruits and veggies (or potatos or sweet potatos). People do very well eating 90% of their calories from starch, and the other 10% from fruits and vegetables.

Starches are plant storage polymers of glucose...

The **Aztecs & Mayans** existed for 9,000 years and were known as people of the corn...

Potatos have been the sustaining food in the Andes of **South America** for 13,000 years...

Wheat and barley was the sustaining food of the **middle east** for thousands of years. The middle east was known as the bread basket of the world...

Asia has primarily eaten rice for the last 10,000 years...

In the **middle east** they've eaten barley and oats for 11,000 years.

In **Africa** they've eaten Millet and Sorghum for 6,000 years.

In the **Near East** they've eaten wheat for 10,000 years, and they're thin; they don't have any "wheat belly or grain brain."

One of the big difference between humans and other primates is that we are designed to digest STARCH. That's why we are able to move away from the equator, but the other primates can't....

Hunter gatherer populations were mostly gatherers... Humans are starchivores... Old school anthropologists overemphasized meat consumptions in early humans, because bone remnants last longer, than plant remnants... 99.9% of all people who have walked on this earth have eaten starch based diets

However, more recent **anthropologist** have been able to study petrified feces from about 600,000 years ago, and they have concluded that early humans ate starch; and that early humans (Neanderthals) ate cooked starch 50,000 years ago...

Cooking dates back over 1 million years. **Brain development** requires an abundance of **carbohydrates**. The brain burns 20% of the calories that we eat, and the brain prefers carbohydrates. Eating cooked starch is what enabled humans to develop the brain power that they have.

You've been told that the agricultural revolution started 10,000 years ago, but in reality, people have been eating starches for hundreds of thousands of years.

Anthropologists have found starch grains in the teeth and feces of other ancient populations from thousands of years ago….

What about the fat vegan? Many of them are eating **nuts and seeds** (80-90% fat) and **avocados** (88% fat) and **olives** (over 90% fat). **You have to avoid these foods if you want to lose weight.**

Eating oil makes you wear oil! You get oily skin, and acne, including from olive oil.

Nuts and seeds are probably the biggest reason for fat vegans.

Dried fruits also contribute to causing obesity, b/c I can eat 20 dried apples in the time it takes to eat 2 regular apples. **Juice** can lead to obesity. You don't improve the quality of a food by making it into a smoothie.

When people want to lose weight, I recommend to **reduce fruit intake** to 1 or 2 servings per day.

Good to also avoid **breads** for losing weight.

If you eat more greens, you will lose weight faster.

Avoiding soy helps you to lose weight.

Do not add **salt**. Salt makes food taste better, and gets you to eat more of it.

Avoid eating out, because they usually put oil in your food. If you actually follow this diet, you will lose weight towards your optimal bodyweight.

The McDougall diet is usually 90% starch, 10% fruits and vegetables. However, when a patient is trying to lose weight, I recommend increasing the amount of vegetables. To lose weight I recommend to decrease starch to 70% of calories, and make 25% of calories come from green & yellow veggies.

The more green and yellow veggies a person eats, the more they will lose weight. A person can eat as much as 50% of calories in the form of green and yellow veggies. But they can't go beyond that. If they try to eat more than 50% of calories in the form of veggies, they won't be able to satisfy their hunger.

Wlater Kempner MD was born in 1903 in Germany. His mentor was Otto Warburg, the great biochemist. Kempner fled Germany in the 1930's, and was able to secure a job at Duke university medical center in North Carolina.

Kempner had done research on kidneys, and thus had a good background for thinking about diets to prevent hypertension and kidney failure.

Walter Kempner MD has an unprecedented record of curing chronic dietary diseases. The drug therapies do not even come close to the results of Dr Kempner. **Kempner's diet was white rice, fruit, fruit juice, table sugar, and vitamins.** The diet consisted of **94% carbohydrate, 4% protein, and 2% fat.**

Fruit and rice chosen because they are very low in sodium. Fruits and vegetables are also very alkaline.

Kempner's diet had an incredibly low sodium content of only about 100 mg/day. This is a very low amount of daily dietary sodium.

It was rare, but for some patients this was too low of a sodium intake, and they were at risk to become sodium depleted; these were patients with the syndrome of inappropriate ADH (SIADH) secretion who could not dilute their urine; also some patients who had had bowel surgery.

[Frank Neelon MD, the doctor who worked with Dr Kempner, said that nowadays, if he was treating patients with the rice diet, he would aim for them to receive about 500-700 mg of sodium per day...

Neelon says that he tries to take patients off blood pressure medications as much as possible. He says that when he is reluctantly obligated to give an anti-hypertensive medication, he tries to give the lowest dose possible.]

Calories were restricted only when weight loss was a goal.

Reference: Newbourg et al. Book. Walter Kempner and the Rice diet. 2011.

The patients had to follow the Kempner rice diet closely, or it doesn't work.

If patients were losing too much weight, he would allow them to eat white sugar to get extra calories. Kempner published a study where he had a group of weight loss patients, 106 of them, who lost an average of 141 lbs, with each of them losing at least 99 lbs.

Beginning in 1944, Ancel Keys (1904-2004), helped with a hunger-starvation study done with Americans, mostly conscientious objectors. It was called the Minnesota Starvation Experiment (MSE).

The 36 men in the study were fed a semi-starvation diet for 6 months at 1, 570 calories per day. All men started trim with "normal" weights. The food served was potatos, turnips, rutabagas, dark bread, and macaroni. There were sufficient calories served to prevent the development of ketosis.

As the partial starvation continued, they became obsessed with food. The felt a decrease in sex drive. All interest in women and dating was lost. They talked about food, read about food, dreamed about food, daydreamed about food.

When they actually were served a meal, they guarded it defensively with their elbows. They ate the food served to them down to the last crumb, and licked their plates clean. Some even became upset when nonparticipants in the cafeteria "wasted" food.

When a person is starving, they only see food.

They commonly had anxiety and depression. They developed extreme tiredness, cold intolerance, muscle soreness, sunken faces & bellies, hair loss. Some lost 33% of their bodyweight = 50 lbs. **Reference:** J bioeth inq Sep 2021; 18(3):407-416.

Most people have a SET POINT for their body weight. If you see them at least once every six months, you will notice that their bodyweight tends to remain the same. On a given diet, the body has a set point for how much that person will eat, and how much they will weigh.

Eating a high fat diet makes the body set point hgh.

Eating a high fat diet with oils tends to increase the set point = makes the person fatter.

After the MSE, the patients underwent 2 months of rehabilitation, where some were allowed to eat unrestricted amounts of food. The interesting thing is that many of them GAINED BACK MORE WEIGHT than their original body weight.

This is called the hyper-hunger overshoot of set point. Ie. they were so hungry, that they ate "too much." It's as if their bodies were saying, "We almost starved to death. We need to gain more weight so that if that ever happens again, we will be better prepared to survive it."

The point is that starvation dieting can lead to weight gain; because the person goes back to the original diet that made them fat in the first place; but now their body has a "fear" of starvation, and they tend to have hyperphagia (overeating), which causes them to increase their set point to a higher bodyweight.

They overshoot their original set point. Ie. they set their new set point to a higher body weight!

Reference: Journal of nutrition, 135, 1347-1352.

Reference: Am j clin nutr, 1997, Mar;65(3): 717-23.

Reference: int j obes (Lond), 2020, Jun; 44(6):1243-1253.

Reference: Obes rev. 2015, Feb; 16 suppl 1:25-35.

After the Minnesota starvation experiment, and the men were allowed to eat, their favorite food was the potato. Potatos were the most hunger satisfying food.

High fat foods do no satisfy hunger well. The person tends to overeat too many calories. "It seems that the body is unable to rapidly detect the high energy density of fatty foods."
Reference: Eur j clin nutr, 1995, Sep; 49(9):675-90.

- From **Why am I fat? & Hunger: why diets, drugs and surgeries fail, & I'm so confused by all of the opposing diets out there! & Dr John McDougall & Dr Frank Neelon discuss the famous "Rice Diet" & the deadly truth about free oils** from Dr McDougall you tube channel.

"In 1973 I changed my diet. I switched from beef to chicken. Then I learned that chicken is about the same as beef. So I switched to fish. Then I learned that fish was about the same. So I ate more dairy. Then I learned that **dairy is basically liquid meat.** So I gave up dairy. Then I learned that **oils were as bad as meat. So I became a low fat vegan.** But a better name for what I am is a **"Starchivore."** - From **Is Dr McDougall just a low fat vegan?** From Dr McDougall you tube channel.

"Pritikin taught pretty much the same thing as I teach. **Walter Kempner and Nathan Pritikin are the truth tellers...**

It's impossible to be too low in fat, in any naturally occurring diet... The Irish starvation protesters lived for 60 days; they burned mostly fat before dying, and only through about 18% of their protein...

America lost the Vietnam war to rice eaters...

The omega 3 blood test is irrelevant... taking vegetable oil or fish oil supplements is a bad idea. The research shows that **fish oil is NOT cardioprotective**... Of any part of diet, vegetable oils are the strongest cause of cancer…

Oil gets everything to stick together in processed food.

The total cholesterol remains the same whether you are fasting or not. I don't remember the best numbers for LDL. It's enough to just go by total cholesterol. I'm an old country doctor, I **just go by total cholesterol.**

Total cholesterol is sufficient, and is not confusing. Sub particles and subfractions of cholesterol measurements add nothing required for me to help care for you. Total cholesterol is what counts! The cost for testing total cholesterol is about $10-40.

William C. Roberts MD, cardiac pathologist said, "The only absolute, unequivocal, independent atherosclerotic risk factor is an elevated serum total or LDL cholesterol."

For practical purposes, cholesterol is only found in animal foods (in significant amounts). Plants can contain tiny, insignificant amounts of cholesterol. Cholesterol is a precursor for synthesis of steroid hormones, bile acids and vitamin D.

The liver is able to make all the cholesterol that the body needs. The liver is also the principle site of cholesterol excretion.

Cholesterol is converted into bile acids, and then excreted into the bile.

In general, all animal foods are about the same. A muscle is a muscle is a muscle…. Whether it flaps a wing, wiggles a tail, or moves a limb.

Whole flaxseed goes largely unprocessed to the colon, so it can be used to treat constipation. When you grind it up, the fats get exposed, and there is increased risk that it will go rancid…

by the time a person goes on dialysis, they've lost over 90% of their kidney function… T

he studies where they say that nuts don't cause weight gain, they were restricting the amount of nuts the people were eating. Nuts are 80-90% fat; they put them in a shell for a reason...

I like eating rice, sweet potatos, and broccoli…

- from Is the fat you eat, the fat you wear? From Dr M YT channel.

I'm the luckiest doctor in the world, because my patients get well.

The McDougall diet is starch >> fruits and veggies, with no animal foods, and no oils. When you remove the animal foods and oils, you remove most of the fat. For patients trying to lose weight they should also avoid high fat plant foods like avocados, coconuts, nuts, seeds, and soy.

With aging, a person does not have to develop obesity, hypertension, diabetes, and coronary artery disease. With the McDougall diet, people don't get those diseases...- Dr John McDougall.

Reference: **Dr McDougall newsletter, April 2004, people – not their words – tell "the carbohydrate story." Includes pictures of rice eaters vs meat eaters.**

Reference: **Dr McDougall newsletter, November 2006, artificial sweeteners are unnecessary and unwise.**

Reference: **Dr McDougall newsletters, October 2006, July 2013, September 2006, June 2010, December 2012. All with information about sugar (or refined carbohydrates).**

Reference: **Dr McDougall newsletter, , December 2008, the fat vegan.**

Chapter 9. **<u>Hypertension</u>**

"A common myth is that the cause of high blood pressure is idiopathic [unknown]…High blood pressure is a symptom of a cardiovascular system that is ill.   **Many doctors will pull out a prescription pad when a patient's blood pressure is more than 140/80.**

But it's better to wait until they have a higher pressure that's sustained like the recommendations of the Cochrane collaboration. Eg. something like **150-160/90-100 mm Hg.** I typically start HTN medications when the pressure is sustained at over 160/100 mm Hg.

Very few people have that high of a pressure on a sustained basis. Transient episodes like this are common, but sustained is not. Normal blood pressure in a patient who is not on medications is about 110/70…

Now you don't want to lower the **diastolic pressure below 85 mm Hg**, because that is associated with decreased perfusion to the brain and heart; this is associated with increased risk of dizziness, falls, dementia, stroke, heart attack and death…

the blood pressure curve has a U-shape. The U-shaped curve means that the risk of cardiovascular events is increased when the BP is too low (due to overtreatment) or too high (due to undertreatment).

The bottom of the U-shaped curve is about 80-85. The goal of treatment is to keep the blood pressure around 150/90. Treatment to below 140/80 is too low. BP above 160/100 is too high. In between these numbers is the sweet spot = 140-160/80-100. Most patients can achieve this goal with diet therapy alone. You do NOT want to overtreat the BP. Lower is NOT better.

The first step is to get a proper measurement of blood pressure.

No coffee. It's good for the patient to measure their blood pressure at home. The cuff should fit properly, small, usual, large. Quiet room, comfortable temperature. No smoking or exercise in the 30 minutes before check blood pressure. Empty the urinary bladder. Take 3 mesurements at 1 minute intervals. Use the average of the last 2 measurements.

Feet flat on the floor.   The patient should be seated with their feet on the floor. Wait about 5-10 minutes after sitting, before check the blood pressure. No talking during and between measurements. Arm bare and resting.

Mid part of upper arm at heart level. The patient should not be talking while the blood pressure is measured. Exercise on a routine basis leads to lower resting blood pressure. Sunshine lowers blood pressure.

The most important factor in causing blood pressure is the food. **The most important cause of**

high blood pressure is dietary fat which causes the blood to sludge [to thicken]. Chronic hypertension is also associated with an increase in atherosclerosis. These atherosclerotic narrowings lead to increased peripheral vascular resistance.

Salt also plays a role in blood pressure, but it's nowhere near as important as dietary fat. **When you lower sodium intake to about 2,300 mg per day, you only get a small reduction in blood pressure, about 3/1 mm Hg**….

Now **if you get real serious about lowering your sodium intake: to less than 500 mg Na+ per day, then you can get profound decreases in your blood pressure.** The McDougall diet typically has about 500 mg sodium per day.

Hypertension should only be treated with medications after it has been sustained for months at 160/100 mm Hg or higher. The best medication for HTN is the diuretic, Chlorthalidone. BP should be lowered to no less than 140/90 with medication.

Usually, I can successfully treat hypertension by diet alone. When I need to use a medicine, I use **chlorthalidone**, (CTD) because it has been shown to reduce the risk of stroke.

Chlorthalidone is a diuretic, but it is NOT the same as hydrochlorothiazide (HCTZ). HCTZ is the most commonly prescribed diuretic in the USA by far. CTD is the only anti-hypertension medication that has been shown to reduce the risk of stroke.

There's a very narrow range of blood pressure for which you should treathypertension. If you look up the papers, you will see that there is darn good reason to choose CTD as the best medicine for treatment of HTN.

References: Treatment blood pressure targets for hypertension (review) of Cochrane database syst rev 2009, Jul 8: by Wright et al. "treating patients to lower than the standard BP targets of 140-160/90-100 does NOT reduce morbidity or mortality."

Reference: British hypertension society guidelines for hypertension management 2004 (BHS-IV): summary, BMJ, 2004, Mar 13;328(7440):634-40. "All people with high BP, borderline or high normal BP should be advised on lifestyle modifications. **Initiate antihypertensive drug therapy if SUSTAINED [means for months] systolic blood pressure > 160 mm Hg or sustained diastolic > 100 mm Hg.**

Reference: JAMA Feb 5, 2014, Vol 311, Number 5, evidence based guidelines for management of high blood pressure in adults by Eduardo Ortiz et al. Says the same thing in more detail.

Reference: Dr McDougall newsletter, March 2004, Take your BP at home, and get off medications.

Reference: **Dr McDougall newsletter, Novermber 2009, How I treat patients with elevated blood pressure.**

Reference: Dr McDougall newsletter, September 2015, patients advised to take more blood pressure pills.

Reference: Dr McDougall newsletter, August 2006, overtreated blood pressure kills.

Reference: Dr McDougall newsletter, July 2004, overtreat your blood pressure, and you could die sooner.

Reference: Dr McDougall newsletter, February 2007, Disease mongering: new women's guidelines for heart disease.

Blood pressure medicines are "poisons" that disrupt normal body functions through chemical reactions. Poisons is the correct word to describe these drugs.

Beta blockers poison the heart muscle. People on beta blockers often complain that they can't walk up stairs because their muscles are so weak.

ACE inhibitors are poisons of the adrenal glands to prevent the production of angiotensin 2. **Angiotensin Receptor Blockers (ARB's)** block angiotensin 2. Doctors often confuse ACE inhibitors and ARB's. Dr's think that these are the same thing. They're not. ARB's might increase the risk of MI. **Reference:** Circulation, 2006, 114: 838-854. ARB's have names that end in "sartan" like LoSartan, ValSartan, etc. I never prescribe ARB's.

Calcium Channel Blockers (CCB's) are poisons, that poison the blood vessels so that they relax. These poisons artificially reduce the perfusion pressure to the heart and the brain, and they increase the risk of dying if you overtreat.

I do not prescribe CCB's for HTN, b/c when CCB's are added to a diuretic, or used alone there is an an **increased risk of myocardial infarction of about 60%.** That doesn't make sense. To try to prevent heart problems by using a drug that increases heart problems.

Reference: Jama, 1995, 274, (8):620-625, Risk of myocardial infarction associated with antihypertensive drug therapies. **CCB's cause constipation. CCB's increase the risk of suicide.**

Reference: Use of CCB's and risk of suicide in population based cohort study. BMJ 1998, 316(7133):741-745. And, **CCB's might increase risk of overall cancer, especially breast cancer.**

Reference: Calcium channel blockade and incidence of cancer in aged populations, Lancet, Aug 24, 1996. There is no reason to use CCB's for treatment of HTN. CCB's include diltiazem, amlopidine, nifedipine. I never prescribe CCB's.

Let's get to the main point. **Sick people take medications; healthy people don't.**

When a patient stops eating high fat diets, their blood pressure drops rapidly.

They need to have their medications reduced or stopped. They are at risk to drop their BP too low. They are at risk for hypotension where they could become dizzy and fall or get into a car accident. It's safer to have a high blood pressure, than too low of a blood pressure. It's easy to teach a doctor how to lower these blood pressure medications when a patient goes low fat vegan.

They should check their BP in the morning, because that's when it's going to be the highest. Sick people take medications. Healthy people do not take medications.

Sick people have surgical scars on their abdomen and chest. Sick people have regular doctor visits. You want to get out of the medical business.

The only way to get out of the medical business is to stop being sick. The only way to stop being sick is to regain your health; to fix the problem. The problem is the food.

The lowering of sodium in the DASH diet trial in 1997 didn't lower BP that much. Eg. lowering sodium intake from 3,000 mg/d to 1,500 mg/d. [Dr Kempner would say that the sodium here is still too high to activate a threshold for significantly lowering BP].

Walter Kempner taught me that diet therapy was the most powerful therapy that there is.

Kempner practiced before anti-HTN drugs were available. Kempner severely restricted sodium, to get daily sodium intakes to below 500 mg/day. **Kempner not only improved the blood pressures, but his diet opened up arteries as indicated by normalization of EKG's in many patients.**

The McDougall diet is effective for lowering blood pressure in hypertension patients. Even after taking 90% of patients off their BP medications, within 7 days the average drop in BP was 18/11 mm Hg. My low fat vegan diet for treatment of hypertension does NOT allow nuts, seeds or avocados. Blood pressure also improves as the person's bodyweight optimizes towards normal.

To determine what is your optimal bodyweight, you can take your clothes off, and look in the mirror. If you like what you see, then your bodyweight is probably okay. You can also look at the recommended bodyweights of Dr Walter Kempner.

- from the **best diet for hypertension** and the **Shocking truths about high blood pressure! Dr McDougall reveals all (part 1)** and **Hypertension: drugs or diet** by Dr McDougall (Dr M) at YT (you tube channel).

Dr McDougall, July 2004 newsletter, Over treat your blood pressure and you could die sooner.

The reason that too aggressive treatment of hypertension with medications causes serious harm is because the artificially lowered blood pressure impairs blood flow to the heart and the brain. This can resullt in heart attack or stroke. Even before the point of heart attack, this can lead to arrhythmias of the heart, which can be fatal.

Overtreated, low blood pressure is associated with poor thinking. Overtreatment of hypertension can lead to dementia.

[**Additonal comments by Peter Rogers MD.** Processed foods are high in sodium. When you stop processed foods, you lower your sodium intake.

Low fat plant foods have addiional features that lower BP. Plants are relatively high in potassium, and low in sodium.

Richard Moore MD, Phd, author of High Blood Pressure solution wrote that it's helpful to have a K factor of at least 5:1. K factor is the ratio of potassium (K+) to sodium (Na+). Our ancestors likely had K factors of over 20:1.

Modern Westerners tend to have K factors of around 1:10. Plant foods are also high in magnesium, because magnesium is located in the center of chlorophyll. Plant greens also tend to be high in nitrates, which are precursors for making nitric oxide. Nitric oxide is a vasodilator, which lowers blood pressure.

Dr McDougall is not that big a fan of magnesium supplements, because he says they can lead to significant side effects.

Plant foods also are contain antioxidants which are helpful to vascular health. Plant foods also contain fiber. The fiber helps prevent leaky gut. Normal gut tight junctions prevent postprandial endotoxemia; this prevents amyloidogenic clotting of the blood. Ie. this prevents RBC's from aggregating; this lowers blood viscosity; this lowers blood pressure.]

Reference: **Dr McDougall newsletter, April 2004, need potassium, take vegetables, not pills.**

Chapter 10. **Diabetes**

"Normal healthy people have good insulin sensitivity. In a healthy person, when insulin binds to the receptor on a cell [like a skeletal muscle cell,] the cell activates glucose transporters [glucose type 4 transporters] to allow glucose to enter the cell.

In **type 1 diabetes,** the patient doesn't have any insulin. Type 1 diabetics do not make insulin, because their pancreas has been damaged by an autoimmune disease, that is associated with eating dairy foods, like cow's milk.

Because they don't have any insulin, they can't get the glucose to go into the cells. This elevates their blood glucose, and is called hyperglycemia. Because they can't get glucose into cells, they become skinny.

For type 1, the patient always needs insulin, or the patient dies. Better for the blood sugar to be high, than to be low. Low blood sugar levels are dangerous. Aggresive therapy to lower blood glucose levels leads to more patients dying."

In **type 2 diabetes,** they've got insulin, often lots of it. Type 2 diabetics tend to have 2x as much insulin as healthy, non-diabetic persons. In type 2 diabetes, the problem is that the insulin receptor is NOT responding to the insulin; this is called insulin resistance. Type 2 diabetics are usually overweight. With type 2, it's always curable with weight loss.

Type 2 diabetes is diagnosed with a finger stick (glucometer) or with blood tests. Normal fasting blood sugar (FBS = Fasting Blood Sugar), is less than 100. Fasting blood glucose greater than 126 mg/dl makes the diagnosis of type 2 diabetes. This threshold of 126, used to be 200. By lowering the FBS number down to 126, lots of new type 2 diabetic patients were "created."

Type 2 diabetes can also be diagnosed by the blood test for hemoglobin A1c (Hba1c). RBC's live about 120 days (3 months). Hba1c is a measure of hemoglobin glycation in RBC's. So hba1c is a measure of glucose control over the previous 3 months.

If Hba1c is over 6.5, that makes the diagnosis of type 2 diabetes. [if hba1c is between 5.5 and 6.5, that makes the diagnosis of Pre-diabetes].

Symptoms of type 2 diabetes include increased urine output, unusual thirst, excess weight loss. Major complications of diabetes include damage to all tissues, especially the eyes, kidneys, nerves, heart.

Type 1.5 diabetes is under recognized. Pt asks "My Hba1c is high, and I'm thin. What should I do? Dr M answers, "You probably have type 1.5, [partial insulin insufficiency diabetes] because you are thin…. Type 1.5 diabetes is also sometimes called partial pancreas insufficiency.

A lot of my patients have type 1.5 diabetes." Type 1.5 diabetics make some insulin, but not enough. Type 1.5 diabetics have enough insulin to avoid getting diabetic ketoacidosis, so they can stay out of the hospital, but not enough to metabolize glucose correctly. Type 1.5 diabetics have partial resistance to insulin. I usually treat type 1.5 diabetes with some insulin so that they don't get too much urine, and thirst.

It has been known for a long time that insulin resistance is caused by a high fat diet.

In 1927, diabetes expert **Elliott Joslin MD** (1869-1962) wrote, "I believe the chief cause of premature atherosclerosis in diabetes, save for advancing age, is an excess of fat, an excess of fat in the body (obesity), and an excess of fat in the diet, and an excess of fat in the blood. With this excess of fat, diabetes begins; and from an excess of fat, diabetics die… of atherosclerosis." **Reference:** Ann clin med 1927;5:1061.

In 1927, **J Shirley Sweeney** took a group of healthy medical students, and fed them two different meals. **Reference:** J Shirley Sweeney, Arch intern med, 1927, 40:818-830. When he fed the students a high carbohydrate diet (sugar, candy, white bread, baked potatos, syrup, bananas, rice, oatmeal), they all tested NORMAL = non-diabetic. When he fed them a high fat meal, they tested positive for diabetes.

[This reminds me of the quote by **Nathan Pritikin,** "All Americans are diabetic after dinner, because they eat high fat dinners. The reason many of them do not test positive for diabetes, is because they are often evaluated in the morning after fasting overnight.]

In 1932, **Dr I. M. Rabinowitch** in Canada wrote about the benefits of high carbohydrate diets for the treatment of type 2 diabetes. **Reference:** Can med assoc j, 1930, 26:142-148. "May I, however, observe that we now have over 500 patients on this diet, and that 16 failures among them, is at least in my opinion, a highly satisfactory state of affairs."

Classic research was done in 1940 by **Himsworth**. **Reference:** Br med J, 1940, May 4; 1(4139):719-22. The same patient was fed two different meals, and their blood glucose was then checked about every 10 minutes for over 3 hours.

After eating a high fat meal (that was low in carbohydrate) the patient had a markedly elevated blood glucose level known as impaired glucose tolerance. When the same patient ate an equicaloric, high carbohydrate-low fat meal, their blood glucose level was much lower; they had improved glucose tolerance.

Reference: Wolpert et al. Dietary fat acutely increases glucose concentration and insulin requirements in patients with type 1 diabetes: implications for carbohydrate based bolus dose calculations and intensive diabetes management. Diabetes care, Nov 27, 2012.

Reference: Brunzell et al, Improved glucose tolerance with high carbohydrate feeding in mild diabetes, NEJM, 1971, mar 11; 284(10):521-4.

Omega 3 supplements worsen type 2 diabetics. **Reference.** elevated plasma glucose and lowered triglyceride levels from omega 3 fatty acid supplementation in type 2 diabetes. By John Ensinck et al. Diabetes care, 1989, Apr, 12(4):276-81. After omega 3 fatty acid supplementation (8 grams per day for 8 weeks) the fasting plasma glucose levels increased 22%… postprandial blood glucose levels increased 35%.

It's better to undertreat type 1 diabetes with insulin, than to overtreat it. If one gives too much insulin, then the patient can become hypoglycemic [blood glucose too low]. Hypoglycemia can cause serious side effects. Hypoglycemia can lead people to thinking and cause them to get a ticket for DUI (Driving under the influence of alcohol).

Hypoglycemia can lead them to getting injured. I try to make things easier for the type 1 diabetic patients. I try to treat them with one injection of a long acting insulin like Lantus or Levemir, etc.

With improved diet, which means switching to a starch based diet, I can typically lower their daily insulin dose by 1/3 to ½. Patients taking insulin medications need to keep a source of sugar around to treat themselves if they get hypoglycemia. Hypoglycemia can cause symptoms like hunger, shaky, sweaty, confused, grumpy, headache, dizzy, etc [scintillating scotoma].

Dietary fat worsens type 1 diabetes. **Reference:** Diabetes care, 36:810-816, (2013). Dietary fat acutely increases glucose concentrations and insulin requirements in patients with type 1 diabetes. Seven patients with type 1 diabetes: high fat dinner required more insulin than low fat dinner (13 vs 9 units).

Before 1980, people in China ate 90% of their calories from white rice, and diabetes was very rare; less than 1% of the population. Nowadays [lecture in 2022], China has become a wealthy country, and they eat a more westernized, higher fat diet. In 2018, the incidence of diabetes in China was 12.4%, and of prediabetes was 50%. **Reference:** Prevalence and treatment of diabetes in China, 2013-2018. JAMA.

Walter Kempner MD (1903-1997) with the Rice Diet, at Duke university in Durham North Carolina cured 100% of his type 2 diabetes patients. The kempner rice diet was 94% carbohydrate, 4% protein, 2% fat. The Kempner rice diet was white rice, fruit, fruit juice, white sugar, and a mulitvitamin.

White sugar was given in larger amounts if the patient wanted it to maintain their bodyweight. He recorded a decrease in heart size and reversal of heart failure in some patients. Kempner recorded hypertensive retinopathy reversal.

Reference: postgrad med, 1958, Oct, 24(4): 359. and

Reference: Am j med, 1959, Au27:196-211. Kempner recorded reversal of obesity, hypertension, and diabetes.

Reference: Am J Med, 1948, 4(4):545-77.

Nathan Pritikin. Nathan Pritikin is my most important mentor. When diabetic patients ate the Pritikin diet, a low fat, plant based diet, at the Pritikin longevity center, their fasting blood glucose decreased a lot, from 183 to 150; and their need for medications was also markedly reduced. **Reference:** J Appl Physiol 2005, Jan, 98(1): 3-30.

The American Diabetes Association diet is relatively high in fat with 40% of calories from fat. Nathan Pritikin said that the ADA diet guarantees that the type 2 diabetic patient will NEVER be cured of type 2 diabetes.

[Dr Rogers went to the store to look at the food recommended for diabetes, expecting then (about 25 years ago) that it would be the healthiest food, because those patients were so sick. Instead, it was a bunch of highly processed, junk food.]

Reference: Curr diab rep 10, 152-158 (2010). the **Adventist health study-2.** The more plant based the person was, the lower the risk of diabetes. Incidence of type 2 diabetes: **nonvegetarian > semi-vegetarian > pesco-vegetarian > lacto-ovo vegetarian > vegan.**

John McDougall MD. For someone eating the McDougall diet, the risk of developing type 2 diabetes is essentially zero%. The McDougall diet has no downside. No adverse effects. No additional costs…. most type 2 diabetics can come off all their diabetes medications within 48 hours of beginning the Mcdougal diet at our facility.

The McDougall diet cure rate for type 2 diabetes is 100%.

It's important for patients to realize that fat causes diabetes. How can a patient get better if they don't know that. If they don't know that, then they don't know what they should do.

Sugar does NOT cause diabetes. Sugar makes diabetes better.

Reference: NEJM 1971, Mar 11; 284(10):521-4. When, over 10 days, fed a diet of 85% carbohydrate (instead of 45% carbohydrate), the FBS (fasting blood sugar) fell, OGTT improved, fasting insulin was decreased. These data suggest that the high carbohydrate diet increased the sensitivity of the peripheral tissues to insulin.

Reference: David Jenkins et al. Type 2 diabetes and the vegetarian diet. Am j clin nutr 2003, Sep; 78(3 suppl) 610s-616s. Improvements in blood sugars in diabetics with 39% stopping insulin, and 71% stopping diabetic pills after 3 weeks of therapy.

Others have also reversed retinopathy with a low fat diet. Like Van Eck. **Reference:** Postgrad med 1958, Oct; 24(4):359-71. and **Reference:** Am J med, 1959, Aug; 27:196-211.

The best diet for diabetics is a low fat, starch based, vegan diet with no oils... Why manage type 2 diabetes with pills, when you can CURE IT with diet?...

French fried potatos are a high fat food, and can cause problems like other high fat foods. However, regular potatos by themselves, when baked or boiled, do NOT cause diabetes. In fact, it's good to feed potatos to diabetics. Potatos only have 1% of their calories from fat.

Low carb diets are a bad idea. The 4 long term studies on low carb diets all show that low carb diets increase mortality. The patients die sooner.

With type 2 diabetes, the oral drugs are dangerous; they can lower blood sugar, but at a price; they kill type 2 diabetics. FDA approval for diabetes drugs is based on their ability to lower blood glucose levels; [it is NOT based on mortality or other relevant health outcomes.] Black women have increased risk of type 2 diabetes, because they tend to eat a poor diet. **Reference:** Trends in lifetime risk and years of life lost due to diabetes in the USA, 1985-2011: a modelling study. Lancet diab endocrinol, 2014, Nov 2(11):867-74.

Diabetes medications can create a vicious cycle; the medications can cause weight gain; then the weight gain can worsen their diabetes. If the patient improves their diet; and eats a starch based vegan diet with no oils, they can typically lose weight, and cure their type 2 diabetes. Some of the newer diabetes drugs can lower cardiovascular risk factors a little, but they cause an increase in other problems. Sulfonylurea drugs were also used as herbicides. Reference: Jama 1971, Nov; 218(9):1400-10.

Intensive medical management of type 2 diabetes is harmful. When type 2 diabetes is overtreated, the outcomes are worse. Hypoglycemia is dangerous. All six studies on aggressive-intensive management of blood glucose levels in diabetic patients shows that this kills more patients. **Reference:** ACCORD study (Action to Control Cardiovascular Risk in Diabetes). NEJM 2008, Jun 12;358(24): 2545-59.

Intensive managmement of type 1 diabetes is harmful. May increase risk of coronary artery disease... more weight gain, higher blood pressure, and higher levels of triglycerides, total cholesterol, LDL, apolipoprotein B. **Reference:** JAMA, 1998, July 8; 280(2):140-146.

Reference: ADVANCE study. Action in Diabetes and VAscular disease. **Intensive blood glucose control** and vasscular outcomes with type 2 diabetes. NEJM 2008, Jun 12;358(24):2560-72. There were no significant effects of this type of glucose control on major macrovascular events, death from cardiovascular causes, or death from any cause... hypoglycemia was more common.

Bariatric surgery can cure obesity, but at a high price. Bariatric surgery is surgically induced malabsorption and sickness. Bariatric surgery can cure type 2 diabetes. Any type of weight loss can cure type 2 diabetes...

Plant based diet can be very helpful for treating painful diabetic neuropathy. The study by Dr **Neal Barnard** showed that a plant diet is a helpful way to treat diabetes. The patients were randomized to a low fat plant based diet for 20 weeks, and they showed a significant reduction in diabetic neuropathy pain.

Reference: Neal Barnard et al. "A dietary intervention for chronic diabetic neuropathy pain: a randomized controlled pilot study." Nutr diabetes, 2015, May; 5(5):e158.

Reference: J of nutritional medicine, 1994, 4, 431-439. Milton G Crane MD and Clyde Sample RD, "Regression of diabetic neuropathy with total vegetarian (vegan) diet." Complete relief of the systemic, distal, polyneuropathy pain in 17 of 21 patients in 4 to 16 days.

With diabetic neuropathy, the number one goal is to cure the type 2 diabetes. Numbness and tingling with diabetic neuropathy can be related to poor blood flow. Low fat vegen diet improves blood flow.

A lot of doctors think that **metformin** is a very good medicine. I'm not convinced.

Reference: reappraisal of metformin efficacy in the treatment of type 2 diabetes: a meta-analysis of randomized controlled trials. Plos medicine april 2012. Although metformin is considered the gold standard, its benefit/risk ratio remains uncertain. We cannot exclude a 25% reduction or a 31% increase in all cause mortality. We cannot exclude a 33% reduction or a 64% increase in cardiovascular mortality." [metformin is a mitochondrial inhibitor.]

Type 1 diabetes is an autoimmune disease that is related to dairy. Everyone should know this about type 1 diabetes.

Reference: NEJM 1992, Jul 30, 327(5):302-7. A bovine albumin peptide as a possible trigger of insulin dependent diabetes mellitus by Hans Michael Dosch et al. Bovine serum albumin (BSA) is the milk protein responsible, and an albumin peptide containing 17 amino acids (ABBOS) may be the reactive epitope.

Antibodies to this peptide react with p69, a beta-cell surface protein that may represent the target antigen for milk induced beta-cell-specific immunity… patients with insulin dependent diabetes mellitus have immunity to cows-milk albumin."

- from **Cure your diabetes with these simple changes** and **How to cure autoimmune diseases** by Dr McDougall at his you tube channel (Dr McDougall Health & Medical Center).

Chapter 11. **Cancer**

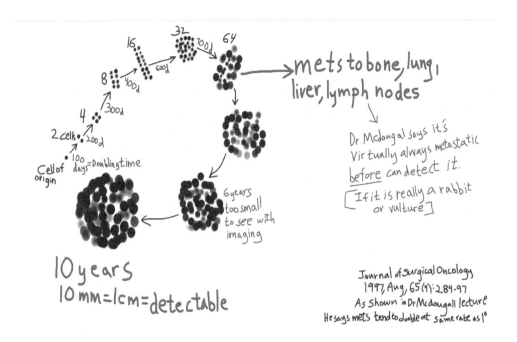

Fig 11-1: "Cancers often double in size about once every 100 days. **Thus the cancer has been there about 10 years before it reaches a detectable size of about one centimeter.** We usually can't see it, or can't confidently call it a cancer, until the tumor is at least one centimeter in size.

[Eg. PET (Positron Emmission Tomography) scans usually can't detect a lung cancer until it is at least about 1 cm in size. When the lung nodule is smaller than 1 cm, it will usually be followed with serial CAT scans, to see whether or not it is growing. Subcentimeter lung nodules are very common, and usually do not grow, but one needs the followup scans to know that for certain.]

If a cancer is going to metastasize, it will usually have metastasized, BEFORE it reaches 1 cm in size. Mets tend to double at the same rate as the primary tumor. This is typical growth.

PSA (prostate specific antigen) doesn't usually become "positive" until the prostate tumor is 1 cm in size.

Mammography detected tumors have usually been growing for about 14-17 years before detected.   The average doubling time for a breast cancer is 100 days. On average, a breast cancer takes 6 years to become 1 mm in size, and 10 years to become 1 cm in size. **By this time, if it is going to metastasize, it probably has already done so.**

The point is that "so called" early detection is really **LATE DETECTION;** ie. after metastasis has already occurred.

This means that local treatments like surgery and radiation are unlikely to cure the patient. Whether the patient lives or dies usually depends on metastases, rather than the primary tumor (with some exceptions, like with brain tumors).

Another key point is that **cancers usually metastasize first to the VEINS, not to the lymph**

141

nodes.

Thus surgical removal of the adjacent lymph nodes usually doesn't do much for prognosis. Those lymph nodes are trying to fight the cancer.

Doctors used to think that cancer spreads primarily through the adjacent lymph nodes. The idea of the centripetal spread of cancer theory suggests that cancer tends to grow outward from a central source; however, that is often incorrect.

In reality, cancer, that's going to metastasize, tends to initially spread through the veins, and can quickly travel to distant sites. Again, this is why local therapies are less effective than was previously thought.

Reference: Br J dis chest 1979, Jan; 73(1):1-17. **Reference:** J surg oncol 1997, Aug;65(4):284-97. AAPS J. 2019, Feb 8; 21(2):27. **Reference:** Cancer. 1961 Nov Dec;14:1272-94. **Reference:** Postgrad med. 17:280-285, (1955).

[Even small **cancers tend to shed a lot of cells into the blood.**

A 1 gram tumor can shed **over a million cancer cells into the blood in one day.**

Immune system is needed to remove cancer cells.

Therefore you want to PROTECT your immune system!

Reference: Quantitation of cell shedding into efferent blood of mammary adenocarcinoma"
Thomas Butler, Cancer Res, March 1, 1975, 35, 3, 512-6
Chemo tends to suppress the immune system.

How is the body going to control the tumor if the immune system is suppressed?

This a major problem with chemo.]

I had a doctor friend who was an oncologist. I asked him to show me a paper that indicates that chemotherapy works for solid tumors.

He never could.

Dietary fat in general, and animal fat (saturated fat) and vegetables in particular is associated with prostate cancer risk. Foods high on the food chain are loaded with cancer causing chemicals. Low fat diets may be beneficial at any point in the course of prostate cancer. **Reference:** Nutrients, (2014) Dec 22; 6(12):6095-109. **Reference:** Int J Cancer. (2008), June 1;122(11):2581-5.

I am convinced that diet has a big effect on prostate cancer, and that the SAD diet tends to make prostate cancer more aggressive.

The American Cancer Society now recommends a plant based diet for patients with cancer: "Prudent diets" high in fruits, vegetables, and unrefined grains, and low in meats, sweets, dairy, and refined grains. Stop pouring gas on the fire.

Cancer screening is over rated, and I do not recommend it. The only real way to prove that a screening study is beneficial is to show in a randomized control trial that it reduces that disease mortality, and all cause mortality.

Reference: Estimated lifetime gained with cancer screening tests. A meta analysis of randomized clinical trials. November 2023.   Jama intern med, (2023);183(11):1196-1203. "The findings of this meta-analysis suggest that the current evidence does NOT substantiate the claim that common cancer screening tests save lives by extending lifetime except possibly for colorectal cancer screening with sigmoidoscopy."

There's two ways you can meet a doctor. #1. You go to the doctor's office [because you have a question or you are sick].

#2. **The doctor comes looking for you.** This is the "business" of screening, of trying to find "early" disease.

Disease mongering is turning people into patients for profit. Screening is one of the most profitable ways to gather up the largest number of customers. This is **DISEASE MONGERING.**

If a doctor is going to go around to healthy people, and tell them that they should have a medical test, that test should have really good research data to support it; evidence that people are truly better off for having had the screening test.

"Monger is a derogatory term for a dealer… Disease mongering is the selling of sickness that widens the boundaries of illness, and grows the markets for those who sell, and deliver treatments. It is exemplified most explicitly by many pharmaceutical industry-funded disease-awareness campaigns… disease mongering turns healthy people into patients…" - Roy Moynihan. Reference: PloS med 2006, Apr; 3(4), e191

So called "improved survival" from screening is usually due to lead time bias. Ie. If under control conditions, a patient develops symptoms from a cancer, when they are 79 years old, and then dies when they are 80 years old, that's a 1 year survival.

If the same patient underwent screening, and was diagnosed with cancer at 70 years old, but still died when they were 80 years old, they now survived the cancer for 10 years. However, screening did NOT change the time of their death!

[Screening assumes the workup and treatment of the cancer will be beneficial. That is NOT always the case. Workups and treatment often have a lot of side effects. Treatments often do not work, but cause side effects. Many early cancers are detected that would NEVER have become symptomatic. Ie. it would have been better to not know about them.]

Peter Gotzsche from the Cochrane collaboration is the world expert on the effectiveness of mammograms. He wrote a book about it called **"Mammography Screening.** (truth, lies, and controversy)."

Gotzsche says that **routine mammograms #1. do NOT save women's lives.** #2. increase the number of women overdiagnosed [whose tumor would not have caused symptoms, and thus they would have been better off not knowing about it.] #3. Increases the risk that a woman will get a mastectomy.

Other pioneers helpd show that mammography is not beneficial including Charles Wright MD, and C. Barber Mueller MD.

[In general, if 2,000 women are screened regularly with mammography for 10 years, then ONE WILL BENEFIT from the screening, and she will avoid dying from breast cancer.

However, 10 healthy women will become cancer patients, and be treated unnecessarily. They are at risk for significant side effects from this treatment.

Furthermore, about 200 women will experience a false alarm.

It therefore no longer seems reasonable to attend for breast cancer screening" – Cochrane collaboration brochure on screening mammography in 2013, issue 6, database of systematic reviews.]

Eight randomized studies of breast cancer screening were performed in women over 50 years of age, and only 2 showed benefits.

Reference: Shapiro study in USA from 1963-1969 for women ages 40-64 years old showed a benefit with 29% reduction in deaths.

Reference: The Health insurance plan of New York showed one less death per year for 7,086 patients screened.

Reference: The Canadian national breast cancer study showed ZERO survival benefit, regardless of the number of mammograms.

Reference: The 2006 cancer screening evaluation unit, institute of cancer research, Sutton UK for patients aged 39-41 years showed no benefit.

Reference: The Anderson study in Malmo, Sweden from 1976-1986 for patients ages 45-69 year old, showed no benefit.

Reference: Roberts study in Edinburgh from 1979-1988 women ages 45-64 showed no benefit.

Reference: Dr McDougall newsletter, January 2004, Mammography is a fraud promoted by industry.

Reference: Rutqvist study in Stockholm from 1981-1985 for women ages 49-64 yo showed no benefit.

["Since the benefit achieved is marginal, the harm caused is substantial, and the costs incurred are enormous, we suggest that public funding for breast cancer screening in any age group is NOT justifiable." - Charles Wright MD and C. Barber Mueller MD.]

Many patients that undergo screening mammography end up over diagnosed. Overdiagnosis is defined as detecting a cancer that would not have caused symptoms in the person's lifetime. **Reference:** Ann intern med, (2023), Sep;176(9):1172-1180.

There are several ways to reduce exposure to estrogens: #1. removal of ovaries. #2. tamoxifen #3. aromatse inhibitors #4. chemotherapy #5. eat a starch based vegan diet with no animal foods #6. filter water. 7. Lose weight. Fat cells make estrogen. When you lose weight, you make less estrogen.

Mastectomy has no advantage over lumpectomy. This was evaluated by a random trial. **Reference:** Twenty year followup of a randomized trial comparing total mastectomy, lumpectomy, and lumpectomy plus irradiation for the treatment of invasive breast cancer. Ann surg, 1970; 172(4):711-32. There was no significant difference in overall survival amont the treatment groups."

Reference: Mastectomy vs lumpectomy. Bernard Fisher (1918-2019) et al. NEJM vol 347, no 16, October 17, (2002).

Reference: Randomized trial. NEJM 2023, Feb 16; 388(7):585-594. Breast conserving surgery with clear excision margins, and adjuvant endocrine therapy. No survival benefit from adding radiation to the breast. There was a higher local recurrence rate in the no radiotherapy group 9.5% vs the radiotherapy group .9%.

Radiotherapy to the breast does not improve survival in breast cancer. **Reference:** Lancet, 2014; 384,999570, 1846.

Chemotherapy for breast cancer is chemical castration. **Reference:** Polychemotherapy for early breast cancer: an overview of the randomized trials. Lancet, 1998, Sep 19; 352(9132):930-42. Postmenopausal breast cancer women do not benefit from chemo, because their ovaries are already gone.

There is ZERO% benefit from screening colonoscopy. Gastroenterologists were very upset by this study, (the NordiCC study), but those are the results. However, sigmoidoscopy appears to be the only type of cancer screening that is beneficial. Sigmoidoscopy only bills for about $200, but colonoscopy bills for about $#,000. Nordic european Initiative on Colorectal Cancer (NordICC), NEJM, Oct 2022, 27; 387 (17):1547. 84,585 patietns. No signficant change in the number of patients who died from the scoped group vs the nonscoped group. A 10 year trial.

If you have a negative colonoscopy, it will take another 15 years to develop cancer, and that will take another 15 years to kill you. Ie. you've got 15 + 15 years before you could die. If anyone is recommending colonoscopy screening for you, you could tell them about this lecture, and show it to them.

The 2016 Canadian guidelines do not recommend colonoscopy for colon cancer screening. **Reference:** CMAJ, 2016, March 15;340-8.

It is reasonable to do a screening flexible sigmoidoscopy between the age of 60 to 75 years old; which appers to reduce mortality from colon cancer by as much as 43%. Can do this only once in life.

Reference: Lancet, 2010, May 8, 375 (9726):1624-33.

Reference: Dr McDougall newsletter, August 2010. Colonoscopy: a gold standard to refuse.

Reference: Dr McDougall newsletter January 2007, complications are common from colonoscopy.

Reference: Dr McDougall newsletter, August 2007, colon cancer patients die faster with western diet.

Reference: "Do physicians understand cancer screening statistics?" Ann intern med, (2012), Mar 6;156(5):340-9. Article says, "Most primary care physicians mistakenly interpreted (1) improved survival and (2) increased detection with screening as evidence that screening saves lives. **Few correctly recognized that only (3) reduced mortality in a randomized trial constitutes evidence of the benefit of screening. To be beneficial, a cancer screening test MUST delay death (reduce overall mortality).**

Prostatectomy surgery is removal of the prostate. Prostatectomy surgery often causes impotence. Prostatectomy surgery for prostate cancer is often unnecessary. In fact, in some studies, there was NO SIGNIFICANT DIFFERENCE between radical prostatectomy and watchful waiting on all cause mortality.

Ie. why have your prostate surgically removed, with all the potential side effects, when the patients who had ZERO surgery did just as well in terms of survival (all cause mortality).

The watchful waiting group (they had no surgery, but could follow their PSA) had less imptence and urinary incontinence. **Reference:** Int j impot res, (2021) May;33(4):401-409.

Reference: JAMA, (2018), May 8;319(18):1914-1931. **Reference:** Iran j public health, (2019), Apr; 48(4):566-578.

I tell my asymptomatic patients that they should not check their PSA. Their's no survival benefit.

With regard to those patients diagnosed with prostate cancer, I recommend watchful waiting to all of them.

Prostate cancer is more common in wealthy countries, because they eat more animal foods, including dairy.

PSA is a high risk test. If the PSA is significantly elevated, typically a prostate biopsy will be recommended. Microscopic prostate cancer is super common. The older the patient, the higher the risk that a random prostate biopsy will be positive for prostate cancer.

For men in their twenties, 8% of prostate biopsies are positive for cancer.

For men in their thirties, 30% of prostate biopsies are positive.

For men in their fifties, 50% of biopsies are positive.

For men in their seventies, 80% of prostate biopsies are positive for prostate cancer.

Ie. LOTS OF MEN have small, asymptomatic prostate cancers that will NEVER cause any symptoms. It's better to NOT KNOW about these.

Prostate biopsy can consist of about 12 needle specimens obtained from the prostate.

55% of men experience pain with prostate biopsies. Some men become impotent just from the prostate biopsy, about 41% temporarily, and then after 6 months, about 15% of men are still impotent. Infection is the most common complication of prostate biopsy. Fluoroquinolone resistant E. coli rates of infectious complications range from .1% to 7%. Sepsis rates range from .3% to 3.1%, depending on antibiotic prophylaxis regimes. **Reference:** J Urol, 2017, Aug; 198(2):329-334.

Reference: J urol 1993 Aug; 150(2 pt 1): 379-85.

Reference: J urol 2004, Oct 172 (4, part 1 of 2):1297-1301.

Reference: J urol 2009, Dec 182(6):2664-9.

Reference: J natl cancer inst 1998, June 17;90(12):925-31.

References: Dr McDougall newsletters about prosate cancer include: April 2004, February 2003, March 2011, March 2010, June 2004, September 2004. May 2008. August 2009. September 2009 No treatment is better for [some] prostate cancer.

Testosterone supplements in men cause increased risk of heart disease. **Reference:** Testosterone treatment and fractures in men with hypogonadism. Nissen et al. NEJM, (2024), Jan 18;390(3): 203-211.

Vaginal estrogen therapy appears to be safe in women with breast cancer. **Reference:** Vaginal estrogen therapy use and survival in females with breast cancer. JAMA oncol, (2024), Jan 1; 10(1):103-108.

Western diet causes earlier onset of puberty, before girls are emotionally ready for that. Bovine Leukemia Virus (BLV) is very common in dairy herds (84%) and common in beef herds (38%). BLV is very similar to Human T-cell Leukemia-Lymphoma virus (H-T-LV). The more cow protein people ate, the higher their risk of a lymphoma death.

Reference: J virol 2022, Dec 19, :e0154222.

Reference: PloS one, 2020, Oct 5; 15(10): e0239745.

Reference: Pathogens, 2020, Dec 18; 9(12): 1058.

BLV seems to be associated with increased risk of breast cancer in humans. Reference: Microb pathog, 2020, Dec; 149:104417.

Reference: Int j environ res public health, 2020, 17, 209.

In 1977, Allan S. Cunningham wrote a great paper. Reference: Lancet, 1976, Nov 27; 2(7996):1184. Cunningham pointed out that overnutrition, especially with protein might be a factor in the pathogenesis (cause) of lymphomas... firstly, lymphomas are more common in upper socioeconomic groups, and othes with high food and high protein intakes... highest with bovine proteins...

Secondly, dietary protein augmentation in rats increases the number of lymphomas which they develop... Burkitt's lymphoma appeared to be due to chronic stimulation by malaria...

Cow's milk causes lymph node enlargement. Lymphomas are more common in Celiac disease. Animal foods are a common source of "cancer viruses."

Diffuse large B-cell lymphoma (DLBCL) accounts for 35% of NHL (Non Hodgkins Lymphoma).

There was a patient with a follicular lymphoma, stage 3a, who underwent a 21 day water only fast at True North Health clinic, and it seems to really help. At 9 month followup, the patient's lymph nodes were nonpalpable, and she remained asymptomatic.

High fat diets, such as occurs from most animal foods, can suppress the immune system. Animal foods are acidic, lack dietary fiber, and lack antioxidants.

"In a this metaanalysis there was strong evidence that indicated that consumption of red meat and processed meat is a risk factor for progression of NHL. There was a strong statistical association between red meat intake, and the risk of DLBCL.

Foods of animal origin are likely to play a role in causing Non Hodgkin's lymphoma and Multiple myeloma. Reference: Asian pac j cancer prev, 2014; 15(23): 10421-5.

Current treatment of DLCBL often involves chemotherapy with the R-CHOP method; 40-50% of patients relapse, and redevelop cancer. The McDougall diet should be a part of cancer treatment.

The more dairy a person consumed, the higher their risk of NHL Eating vegetables reduces the risk of getting lymphoma.

- from video **"Dr McDougall's expert guide to beating prostate cancer & surprising facts about estrogen, diets, and cancer"** – by Dr John McDougall from his you tube channel "Dr McDougall Health & Medical Center."

"The more carbohydrate a population eats, the less cancer they have.... If a cancer patient improves their diet, they are likely to live longer... eating sugar doesn't increase cancer, but eating fat does..." – Dr McDougall from "Does sugar feed cancer.

Dr McDougall, newsletter, February 2015, dietary mechanisms for cancer.

1. Losing weight. Obesity increases the risk of getting cancer, and obese people die sooner

from their cancers.

2. Cut out meat. This removes substances known to cause cancer progression.

3. Stop cow's milk. This removes substances known to cause cancer progression.

4. Reduce intake of growth stimulants: Animal foods of all kinds increase growth factors (IGF-1, etc) for cancer progression.

5. Give up vegetable oils: isolated corn, safflower, olive, etc oils will encourage tumors to grow faster (than do animal fats).

6. Avoid cancer promoting chemicals (environmental carcinogens and persistant organic pollutants).

7. Increase immune system enhancing plant components called phytonutrients.

8. Grow healthy intestinal bacteria to enhance the body's defences against cancer.

9. Increase intake of anti-cancer plant sterols.

10. Raise the consumption of cancer fighting folates. As the root word "foliage" implies, these substances are from plants.

Dr McDougall newsletter, December 2006, Raw food vegetarian diet [helps] protect us from cancer.

Dr McDougall newsletter, december 2012. Annual physical exam.

Avoid annual physical exams. The annual physical exam is an intensive, well orchestrated experience designed to make people who are apparently well, be diagnosed as sick (with good intentions). You walk into your doctor's office as George of Francine, and you leave as a patient with a disease.

The main reason detecting disease early does not help reduce death, suffering, and/or disability is that the treatments (pills and surgeries) are ineffective and dangerous.

Dr McDougall newsletter, February 2015, will a healthy diet stop or slow most cancers?

Chapter 12. **Autoimmune disease and Inflammatory Arthritis**

"Upon switching to the McDougall diet, patients will usually start noticing a benefit in about 4-7 days. It takes that long to get the old food out of the colon.

They should expect to improve. The acuity of joint symptoms should decrease. The existing fibrosis in the joints does not go away, but it does not progress.

Within 4-6 months, patients with rheumatoid arthritis, lupus, and psoriasis are often cured.

If the patient does not see significant improvement by 4 months, then they are not going to improve with the McDougall diet alone.

They can consider the more restrictive, elimination diet." - John McDougall MD.

Dr McDougall, newsletter, June 2006. Gout is on the rise.

"The main cause of elevated blood uric acid and gout, is eating animal foods like meat, poultry, fish, and seafood; these are the most important sources of purines. The purines lead to elevated blood uric acid. Vegetable sources of purines do NOT contribute to the risk of having an attack of gout. Alcohol is also believed to encourage the deposition of uric acid crystals in the joints.

When people lose weight, they can get a transient increase in blood uric acid, leading to an episode of gout. This happens because of the body dissolving body fat. The risk of these attacks is very small. One can make a definitive diagnosis of gout by extracting fluid from a painful joint, and putting it under a microscope to show uric acid crystals."

"Here's a list of autoimmune diseases:

Addison's disease (of adrenals)

Alopecia (hair loss) [the mastering diabetes guy has this]

Ankylosing spondylitis (associated with HLA B-27)

Asthma

Reference: Dr McDougall newsletter, May 2010, better breathing from diet.

Celiac disease

151

Crohn's disease

Dermatomyositis

Diabetes type 1

Eczema

Hyperparathyroidism (is probably an autoimmune disease related to overstimulation of the parathyroid glands trying to compensate for excessive dietary intake of phosphates from animal foods). A chronically overstimulated parathyroid gland, can become autonomous, and cause hyperparathyroidism.

Inflammatory arthritis

Interstitial cystitis (inflammation of the urinary bladder) appears to be an autoimmune disease. Please see the **May 2014, McDougall newsletter.**

Juvenile rheumatoid arthiritis

Lupus – Lupus was very rare in Africa where they ate plant based diets. Lupus is relatively common in black American women, who eat very little plant food.

Multiple sclerosis = Roy Swank MD has the best outcomes in the world for treating MS.

Reference: **Dr McDougall newsletter, July 2012, MS drugs are criminally expensive failures.**

Myasthenia gravis

Non specific arthritis

Parkinson's disease is possibly an autoimmune disease, and possibly occurs with increased frequency in multiple sclerosis patients.

Reference: Parkinson's disease and other diet induced tremors in **Dr McDougall Newsletter, November 2010.**

Pernicious anemia

Polymyositis

Psoriasis = skin lesions = typically improves with vegan diet. Kempner reported helping a lot of these patients.

Psoriatic arthritis

Reiter's syndrome

Relapsing polychondritis

Rheumatoid arthritis = typically improves with McDougall diet. Dr McDougall has testimonials at Dr McDougall dot com who had dramatic improvement with the vegan diet. Leaky gut appears to be the main cause of rheumatoid arthritis. RA patients who switch to the McDougall diet usually experience dramatic improvement. RA did not exist anywhere in the world before 1800. RA was very rare in Africa before 1957… After 20 years with RA, the typical patient is disabled or dead, if treated with meds. Avoiding gluten and soy can also help patients to improve from inflammatory arthritis. The worst food; the food most likely to make RA worse is dairy...

Reference: Dr McDougall newsletter, December 2014, Rheumatoid arthritis and meat.

Reference: Dr McDougall newsletter, May 2014, Ten cases of severe, mostly rheumatoid arthritis cured by the McDougall diet.

Schizophrenia is possibly an autoimmune disease. The global distribution of schizophrenia parallels the western diet, diabetes, and coronary artery disease; suggesting that it might be at least in part a dietary disease, and possibly an autoimmune disease. Malcom Peet wrote a paper about this in the British Journal of psychiatry in May 2004. The western diet is also associated with increased risk of depression. **From the August 2004 newsletter by Dr McDougall with article on how the western diet is a cause of schizophrenia and depression.**

Scleroderma

Thyroiditis eg. Grave's or Hashiomotos

Ulcerative colitis

Reference: Dr McDougall newsletter, November 2004, Ulcerative colitis relapses with meat and beef.

Uveitis

Vitiligo

The 1978 **arthritis foundation** put out a **brochure** that said, "There is no special diet for arthritis. No specific food has anything to do with causing arthritis. And no specific diet will cure it. Food fanatics and peddlers of "health" and natural foods may tell you otherwise." Well, I (Dr McDougall) am here to tell you otherwise! This brochure is wrong. The science shows otherwise.

Everyone knows that a high meat diet causes gout. If you look at Asians and Africans **where they eat plant based diets,** osteoarthritis (degenerative joint disease = **DJD) is rare.** Why is osteoarthritis rare in people in Asia and Africa who do heavy labor, but relatively common in Americans, including those who do not heavy labor. It's the food. In my **May 2014 newsletter** I wrote about the role of diet in arthritis…

Some researchers believe that rheumatoid arthritis did not exist anywhere in the world before 1800. **Inflammatory arthritis was once rare or nonexistent in rural populations of Asia and Africa. As recently as 1957, no case of rheumatoid arthritis could be found in Africa.** Whereas nowadays in the USA, the blacks have the highest incidence of lupus [which is associated with arthritis]…

Up until 1980, about 90% of the diet in Asia was rice.

Prior to 1980, less than 1% of Chinese had diabetes; now [in 2013] 11.6% had diabetes, and 50% were prediabetic… **Reference:** Controlled trial of fasting and one year vegetarian diet in rheumatoid arthritis by Hovi, Lancet, vol 338, 1991. The patients on a plant based diet all improved… There's no money to promote this diet.

Some researchers believe that RA did not exist anywhere in the world before 1800. **Reference:** Arthritis rheum 34;248, 1991.

Reference: "McDougall study on RA," by McDougall, J altern complement med, 2002, Feb; 8(1)… The first step to getting inflammatory arthritis is to get leaky gut [increased intestinal permeability]… For people with true celiac disease their intestinal lining can be injured by wheat, barley, and rye…

To get well, the patient should follow the McDougall diet EVERY DAY. If they don't follow the diet, the autoimmune disease can come roaring back in dramatic fashion, (McDougall's revenge), usually within 24 hours. Small amounts of offending foods can cause big reactions. These usually resolve in 4 to 7 days with elimination of the food from the bowel and body.

Dietary fat has a toxic effect on the intestine in experimental animals causing leaky gut… Feeding high cholesterol diets also increases the risk of leaky gut…

Diets high in vegetable oils are known to damage intestinal integrity...

Leaky gut can lead to abnormally big chunks of protein crossing the intestine lining. The immune system makes antibodies to it. These proteins are similar in sequence to that of proteins in our own body. This can lead the antibodies to cross react with our own bodies = to attack our own body, and cause inflammatory arthritis and autoimmune disease..

For example, the residues of bovine albumin #141-157 are highly homologous to those of human collagen, and this is thought associated with rheumatoid arthritis. **Reference:** Clin chim acta, 1991, dec 16, 203(2-3):153-65...

Rheumatoid arthritis is a very serious disease. After 20 years, 35% of the patients are dead. At 20 years, of those still living, 19% are severely disabled. **Reference:** Lancet, 1987, May 16; 1(8542):1108-11.

There are lots of autoimmune diseases including autoimmune alopecia (hair loss), ankylosing spondylitis, Crohn's disease, diabetes type 1, Lupus, MS, psoriasis, scleroderma, rheumatoid arthritis, juvenile RA, thyroiditis, ulcerative colitis, uveitis, vitiligo... Obesity is associated with increased risk of inflammatory arthritis...

Autoimmune diseases have a characteristic **worldwide distribution;** they are more common in **Northern areas**, because the farther one goes from the equator, the **more meat and dairy,** people tend to eat. This is true for **type 1 diabetes,** and many other autoimmune diseases.

In Africa, before 1960, there was no known lupus. Nowadays, in the USA, black women have the highest incidence of Lupus.

In Africa, rheumatoid arthritis used to be very rare. **Reference:** South Africa medical journal, "Rheumatic disorders in the South African Negro," July 26, 1975, vol 49. By 1975, RA was becoming more common in urban areas, and more severe in urban areas, than in rural areas.

Around 1960, the neurologist Roy Swank MD went to China, and the Chinese didn't have any patients that definitely met the diagnostic criteria for multiple sclerosis.

When multiple sclerosis patients ate the McDougall diet for one year, they noticed a significant improvement in fatigue, and showed trends for improvement in mental health quality of life over the one year duration in comparison with controls. **Reference:** McDougall study on fatigue in multiple sclerosis.

After the age of 4 years old, 75% of the world's population can't digest **milk.**

With milk, when the amount of fat is reduced, then the percent of calories from protein and lactose is increased. Whole milk is about 49% fat, and 30% carbohydrate (with percentages here referring to % of calories). Skim milk is about 0-2% of calories from fat, and 57% from lactose.

Milk is associated with a lot of diseases: type 1 diabetes, childhood kidney damage with membranous nephropathy, obesity, constipation, atherosclerosis, osteoporosis, kidney stones, diabetes, multiple sclerosis, coronary artery disease, cataract, etc. Pasteurization does not kill bovine leukemia virus or mad cow disease.

[Mad cow disease is super rare. I've seen two cases in the last 30 years. In comparison, I see obesity, hypertension, diabetes, coronary artery disease, stroke, and cancer, all day long, every day.]

Cataracts are associated with increased dietary meat, dairy, high total dietary fat intake, high cholesterol dietary intake, aging, past eye surgery, diabetes, steroid medications, trauma to the eye, [some contact lens preservatives]. **Reference:** Int opthalmol, 2014, Feb; 34(1):59-68.

The galactose from milk is associated with increased risk of cataracts. Even if a person has lactase enzyme to split the lactose into glucose and galactose; that doesn't meant that they are able to adequately metabolize the galactose. They might accumulate galactitol in the lens which increases their risk of senile cataracts.

I believe that cow's milk is the most common cause of cataracts.

Reference: "Does milk have a cataractogenic effect? Weighing of clinical evidence. Sharma et al. Dig dis sci 1989, Nov; 34(11):1745-50.

Reference: High frequency of lactose absorbers among adults with idiopathic senile and presenile cataract in a population with a high prevalence of primary adult lactose malabsorption. Rinaldi et al. Dig dis sci, 1982, Mar; 27(3):257-264. These results suggest that adults able to absorb the galactose are especially susceptible to senile or presenil cataracts.

Reference: Galactose can cause cataracts. "Galactokinase deficiency and galactosemia." Galactose byproducts are toxic to the eye lens. J am coll nutr, 1991, Feb, 10(1):79-86.

Reference: the journal of nutrition, 1935; 9(1):37-49. Cataracts.

Reference: Br J opthalmol, 1953, Nov;37(11) 655-60. Cataracts.

Drinking milk increases ILGF-1 by an average of 10%. **Reference:** BMJ 1997; 315:1255-1260.

Reference: J am diet assoc 1999; 99:1228-33.

Drinking cow's milk is associated with increased risk of kidney damage called early childhood membranous nephropathy due to cationic bovine serum albumin. **Reference:** NEJM 2011, Jun 2, 364, (22), 2101-10. All four children with circulating bovine serum albumin related membranous nephropathy underwent a complete or partial remission.

Thyroid disease: Two of the most common thyroid diseases are Hashimoto's thyroiditis, and Grave's disease (Thyrotoxicosis).   Hypothyroidism is most often due to autoimmune disease.

A hot dog is a ground up animal, and it contains some thyroid. With leaky gut, some of this animal thyroid can get across the gut lining, and into our blood. Our human immune system recognizes the animal thyroid as foreign, and makes antibodies to it.

The animal thyroid tissue has enough difference to our self, to be recognized as foreign, and to elicit an immune response. However, the shape of the animal thyroid tissue is similar enough to ourselves, that the our own antibodies, can bind to our own thyroid, and "think" it's the foreign protein, and destroy it.

This mechanism is called antigen mimicry (by the foreign protein), with auto-antibody (our own antibody), attacking ourselves (cross reactivity). This is because the sequence of amino acids in animal mammal thyroid tissue, can be similar to the amino acid sequence in our own thyroid tissue.

This mechanism of molecular mimicry with autoantibody cross reactivity is thought to be the mechanism of the most common type of thyroiditis in humans like Hashimoto's thyroiditis.

Once the thyroid is damaged, the damage is usually permanent. The best treatment for hypothyroid is usually the drug called synthroid.

Some patients benefit from avoiding gluten. Celiac disease (CD) is the ultimate in sensitivity to gluten. Celiac disease affects 1% of population or fewer.

High gluten containing foods ae especially rye, barley, and wheat. Starches low in gluten include potatos, sweet potatos, rice, millet, quinoa, etc.

Reference: "Improvement of inflammation and pain after three months exclusion diet in rheumatoid arthritis patients." Nutrients, 2021, 13, 3535. Long standing, well controlled RA. The following foods were excluded: meat, gluten, lactose (all dairy). Duration of 3 months. **Result: better control of inflammation.**

Reference: McDougall study on rheumatoid arthritis. "Effects of a very low fat, vegan diet in subjects with rheumatoid arthritis." John McDougall et al. J altern complement med, 2002, Feb, 8(1):71-5.

Reference: Controlled trial of fasting and one year vegetarian diet in rheumatoid arthritis. Lancet, vol 338, issue 8772, pp 899-902, Hovi et al. "This dietary regimen seems to be a useful supplement to conventional medical treatment of rheumatoid arthritis."

Vegan diet often alleviates the symptoms of fibromyalgia. **Reference:** Scand J rheumatol 2000; 29:308-313. BMC complementary and alternative medicine. Fibromyalgia syndrome improved using a mostly raw vegetarian diet. An observational study.

Schizophrenia is also a western disease. I think that **Schizophrenia is likely an autoimmune disease.**

Reference: Hidden role of gut microbiome dysbiosis in schizophrenia: antipsychotics or psychobiotics as therapeutics? Shizophr res 2016, September; 176(1): 23-35.

Reference: Neurosci biobehav rev 2020, Jan; 108:712-731.

Reference: Schizophrenia: Prog Neuropsychopharmacol biol psychiatry, 1996, Oct; 20(7): 1083-114.

Some autism is also likely due to autoimmune disease.

Reference: Autism: J dev behav pediatr, 2006, Apr; 27 (2 suppl): s162-71.

The McDougall diet is able to cure the majority of patients with autoimmune disease. Usually the patient will know within four months if the McDougall disease can cure them; and by cure I mean stop the disease from progressing. It's not going to restore damaged joints back to normal.

However, in some patients, the McDougall diet is not able to stop the progression of autoimmune disease. In these patients, an elimination diet can be helpful.

Starches allowed with the elimination diet include brown or white rice, puffed rice, sweet potatos, tapioca rice flour, Taro (or poi), winter squash. For more information see the May 2014 newsletter at Dr McDougall dot com.

Fruits allowed with the elimination diet include apricots, bananas, berries, cherries, papaya, peaches, plums, jack fruit, bread fruit.

Veggies allowed with the elimination diet include non-starchy green and yellow vegetables (all **cooked**): asparagus, artichoke, beets, beet greens, celerey, chard, kale, lettuce, string beans, spinach, summer squash.

Cooking a food helps to denature the proteins, which makes the food less likely to elicit an autoimmune response.

Cooking also makes a food more sweet, taste better, because it frees up the simple sugar component. This is also what happens when making juice or a smoothie; the simple sugar component is partially freed up from the adjacent fiber, etc.

The ultimate elimination diet is fasting. The True North health center is well known for helping people with water fasting. Fasting can work very well, but fasting is only a temporary cure. Eventually, a person must eat.

- from the videos **Inflammatory arthritis & How to cure autoimmune diseases & my body is attacking itself! How to cure autoimmune diseases by** Dr John McDougall (Dr M) YT (you tube) channel.

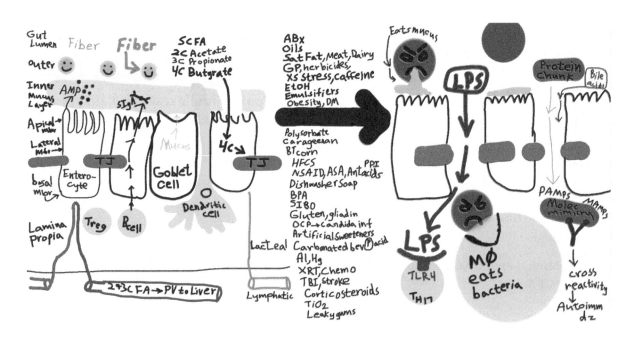

[Fig 12-1: **Normal gut lining** is maintained by eating dietary fiber. Good gut bacteria use dietary fiber to make short chain fatty acids (SCFA), including butyrate.

Butyrate is used by the enterocytes to make tight junctions. Lack of dietary fiber leads to lack of butyrate, leads to loss of tight junctions.

Loss of tight junctions leads to abnormally large chunks of animal protein being able to get across the intestinal lining; and this can cause a big immune system response.

This can lead to molecular mimicry of our own proteins, and autoantibody cross reactivity: ie. our own antibodies attacking our own bodies = autoimmune disease.

Jeff Nelson at Veg source you tube channel says that the McDougall diet cured his daughters of acne, and cured his wife of the autoimmune disease called relapsing polychondritis.

159

When I was young, in my 20's, my girlfriend's mother died of lupus. They had asked me for advice. At that time, I was just a medical student. I didn't have any useful knowledge. I just told them to try to find the best rheumatologist. Her mom was a super nice lady. Oh, how I wish I had discovered Dr McDougall's books at a younger age!]

Dr McDougall, newsletter, January 2014, smoke and mirrors behind Wheat Belly & Grain Brain.

Low carb diets contribute to higher risk of disease and death: 3 studies listed. Animal foods cause inflammation, not plant foods. 6 studies listed.

Why do animal foods cause inflammation:

1. high fat and cholesterol = blood sludge, mild tissue hypoxia, insulin resistance, [increased blood viscosity, MPO (myeloperoxidase) induced collapse of endothelial glycocalyx, etc.]

2. TMAO

3. autoimmune disease

[4. post prandial endotoxemia with amyloidogenic clotting due to LPS and LTA bacterial endotoxins.]

Dr McDougall newsletter, March 2013, Gluten free diets are harmful for the general population (except for one percent).

The current gluten-free diet craze is unhealthy for those who do not need it – those without celiac disease.

Wheat can be associated with celiac disease, wheat allergies, and wheat sensitivity.

Gluten free can be a disguise for low carb eating.

Gluten free diets cause weight gain.

Dr McDougall newsletter, September 2010, Glucosamine and Chondroitin do not help arthritis.

Dr McDougall newsletter, April 2004, how to prevent and treat degenerative (osteo) arthritis.

Chapter 13. <u>Heart disease</u>

"Kempner showed plant based dietary reversal of coronary artery disease by EKG in the 1940's;

Pritikin showed it in the 1960's.

Blankenthorn showed it by cardiac cath in the 1970's;

Ornish showed it in the 1990's.

The ability to partially reverse coronary artery disease with a plant based diet has been known for a long time." - John McDougall MD.

" 4 of 4 studies showed more deaths in the patients eating **low carb diets.**

References: #1. The animal **low carbohydrate** score was associated with **higher all cause mortality** [ie. with pt's eating low carb, more died]. Ann intern med, 2010, Sep 7; 153(5):289-98.

#2. Low carbohydrate high protein diets used on a regular basis… are associated with **increased risk of cardiovascular disease**. [ie. with pt's eating low carb, more died]. BMJ, 2012, Jun 26;344:e4026.

#3. Low carb diets (LCD) were associated with a significantly **higher all-cause mortality.** (Dr McDougall said, "Do you get it? **Low carb diets kill people!**). Plos one, 2013, 8(1):e55030. #

4. Greater adherence to LCD high in animal sources of fat and protein was associated with **higher all-cause mortality** post MI. [ie. with pt's eating low carb, more died]. J Am Heart assoc, 2014, sep 22;3(5):e001169…

#5. Low carbohydrate diets, low fat diets, and mortality in middle aged and older people. 371, 000 patients. **The low fat diet lowered mortality by 18%**. J intern med, 2023:00:1-13.   Dr McDougall says that **Dr Mercola gave up on low carb diets because of this**…

Nowadays they've got drug eluting stents that have chemotherapy like drugs that stop the arterial wall from hypertrophying. All 15 studies show the same thing on percutaneous coronary artery intervention (**PCI**) that there is ZERO reduction in risk of dying.

The other possible treatment is **CABG** (coronary artery bypass graft) surgery, and three studies were done, and they showed **no improvement in survival,** except for a few patients who were very, very sick.

Another study came out, a fourth study, and it showed about the same thing… the low fat diet can stop chest pain, and help arteries to heal… recent data shows that **statins are not that useful**

for reducing the risk of dying from heart disease. They are ineffective. - from **Do low carb diets increase the risk of heart disease** from Dr McDougall (Dr M) YT (you tube) channel.

"The differential diagnosis **(ddx) for chest pain** is esophagitis (pain on swallowing), costochondritis (pain 2 inches from the sternum), pericarditis (outer lining around heart), [myocarditis (heart muscle inflammation), Boerhaave's esophageal rupture (very rare), thoracic aorta dissection (rare), pulmonary embolism, peumonia with pleuritis (rare)].

Angina pectoris (ischemia of heart that is brought on by physical activity or emotional upset. Duration of minutes. Relief follows a short period of rest. Annually, 4% of cardiac angina patients die.

Heart attack = myocardial infarction (MI) = occlusion of a coronary artery which causes heart muscle to die. MI is associated with chest pain, that often radiates into the jaw and/or the left arm. Patients sometimes describe a chest pressure that's like "an elephant sitting on their chest." About 12% of MI do not have little if any chest pain.

In the Western world, the older the patient, the more likely they will have significant coronary artery blockages on an angiogram.

30 yo = 26%.

36 yo = 41%.

40 yo = 53%.

44 yo = 65%.

50 yo = 73%.

55 yo = 79%.

60 yo = 84%.

65 yo = 88%.

70 yo = 91%.

[in other words, if ate the SAD diet, by the time they reach 40 years of age, the majority of persons will have significant blockage at cardiac cath. You don't need to do a screening CT. You need to eat a low fat, starch based, whole food, vegan diet with no oils!]

163

One can also correlate the patient's cholesterol level with the likelihood that they will have a greater than 50% stenosis (stenosis means narrowing or partial blockage), in their coronary arteries. For patients UNDER the age 40 year based on blood total cholesterol level.

Total cholesterol level (mg/dL)	% with positive coronary angiogram
< 200	20
201-225	38
226-250	48
251-275	60
276-300	77
301-350	80
> 350	91

Reference: Circulation, 1970, Oct; 42(4):647-52.

To convert total cholesterol from mg/dl to IU, can divide by 38.

Elevated blood cholesterol is a risk factor, not a disease. You can get a blood test for total cholesterol for only about ten dollars. It is true that sometimes aperson has a high cholesterol, but clean arteries, or even the opposite; a relatively normal cholesterol but has atherosclerosis, but that is not common.

The clinical goal is to get total cholesterol below 150, because persons below 150 have a very low incidence of coronary artery disease. To be below 150 is the ideal level of total blood cholesterol.

Inflation of a balloon in a coronary artery is called balloon angioplasty. The medical abbreviations are **PTCA** (Percutaneous TransCatheter Angioplasty) or **POBA** (Plain Old Balloon Angioplasty). Coronary artery balloon angioplasty was invented by Andreas Roland Gruntzig, a German doctor. Gruntzig encountered obstacles to practice in Germany, so he moved to Switzerland.

Cardiologists started performing balloon angioplasty in the coronary arteries in the late 1970's, but they ran into the problem of distal embolization of atherosclerotic plaque. Ie. pieces of the atherosclerotic plaque would break off the arterial wall, and travel distally to plug up smaller heart arteries.

Then the cardiologists developed bare metal stents **(BMS)** to smoosh the atherosclerotic plaque against the arterial wall. [A BMS is like a soda pop can cylinder with the top and bottom cut out. The walls of a BMS are porous like a chain link fence with only small holes.]

One of the biggest problems with the BMS is that the arterial wall continues to proliferate, [to grow into the stent] and this can occlude the stent. With bare metal stents, about 40% of arteries are closed down within one year.

Then the cardiologists developed a drug eluting stent **(DES).** The DES contains drugs that are like chemotherapy. The drugs dissolve out of the stent, and go to the arterial wall, to prevent it from proliferating.

The DES drug prevents the arterial wall from proliferating. However, the DES chemo drug only lasts about 4 months. The patient is also put on a blood thinner drugs to help prevent the blood from clotting. Typical oral drug therapy to prevent clotting is Dual AntiPlatelet Therapy **(DAPT)** of aspirin and plavix. DAPT reduces the risk of coronary artery clot formation, but increases the risk of bleeding elsewhere.

Placement of stents from a percutaneous approach is usually done by entering the right common femoral artery in the groin area. Placement of a stent into the coronary arteries is called **PCI** (Percutaneous Coronary Intervention). The billing for placement of a coronary artery stent is about $30,000.

Coronary artery stenting has remained very popular for decades because it is:

 #1 profitable.

#2. Seems upon superficial inspection to make sense, as a "logical" treatment.

#3. It's fun to perform for the interventional cardiologist. They tend to enjoy doing these procedures.

#4. The patients are in a sense kind of "self-referred," ie. from one cardiologist to another cardiologist.

#5. the public assumes that all doctors are the same, and that they are in good hands.

In reality, the results of PCI are surprisingly variable. Reference: Circulation volume 67, no.

3:483, (1983). An official journal of the American Heart Association. "Coronary arteriography and coronary artery bypass surgery: morbidity and mortality in patients 65 years or older. A report from the coronary artery surgery study."

If a person has chest pain (CP) that might be a heart attack, they should immediately go to the emergency room. If a cardiologist performs PCI within 90 minutes of CP onset, they can often reopen the artery, and save the patient's life. Even within 6 hours of onset, they can potentially reopen the artery and save a significant amount of cardiac muscle.

The problem with coronary artery stents is that they don't work for the very common problem of cardiac angina with coronary artery atherosclerotic stenosis.

Reference: JACC Cardiovasc interv, 2016, Mar 28;9(6):530-8. Hyung Lee et al. "Successful recanalization of native coronary total occlusion is not associated with improved long term survival." Successful PCI vs failed PCI procedure was not associated with lesser risk for mortality.

Reference: NEJM (2006), Dec 7;355(23):2395-407. "Coronary intervention for persistent occlusion after myocardial infarction." The Occluded Artery Trial (OAT). PCI did not reduce the occurrence of death, reinfarction or heart failure, and there was a trend toward excess reinfarction during 4 years of followup.

Reference: Circ cardiovasc interv, (2012) Aug 1; 5(4):476-90. "Percutaneous coronary intervention vs optimal medical therapy in stable coronary artery disease. A systematic review and metaanalysis of randomized clinical trials. Pursnani et al. 7,182 patients studied. [that's a lot!]. PCI compared with OMT (Optimal Medical Therapy) showed that PCI did NOT reduce the risk of mortality, cardiovascular death, nonfatal myocardial infarction, or revascularization.

CABG (coronary artery bypass graft) surgery is open heart surgery for treatment of atherosclerosis in the arteries of the heart. CABG is an absolute failure, because it treats the wrong lesion. CABG treats the hard, fibrous, NON-LETHAL plaques (scars) which NEVER kill you.

The cardiologist and cardiac surgeon cannot see the tiny, volatile plaques (pustules) that actually, eventually rupture, and kill heart muscle. The culprit lesions, the ones that might actually progress to occlude a coronary artery, are LEFT UNTOUCHED. That's why CABG does NOT prolong life (except under rare circumstances).

The three big studies (and there's only these three big studies) on heart surgery, CABG, show that it lacks survival benefits:

Veterans study 5 year survival rates for surgery = 82%, medical therapy 80%.

European study 5 year survival for surgery 93%, for medical therapy 85%.

CASS study 5 year survival for surgery 95%, for medical therapy 92%. An one must remember that the surgery comes with great financial cost, pain, suffering, risk of complications and death.

Reference: NEJM, "Eleven year survival in the Veterans administration randomized trial of coronary bypass surgery for stable angina." NEJM 311:1333, (1984). Survival among patients with implaired left ventricular function differed significantly at 7 years, but not at 11 years.

Reference: NEJM. "Twelve year followup of survival in the randomized European coronary surgery study. NEJM 319: 332, 1988. The benefit of surgical treatment tended to be greater, but notsignificantly so… the reasons for the loss of a beneficial effect of surgery after 5 years are unknown, and merit further study.

Reference: Circulation, 82: 1629. 1990. Ten year followup of survival and myocardial infarction in the randomized coronary artery surgery study. There were no significant differences either in survival and freedom from nonfatal myocardial infarction, whether stratified on the presence of heart failure, age, hypertension, or number of vessels diseased.

Reference: Circulation 91: 2325, (1995). "Comparison of surgical and medical group survival in patients with left main coronary artery disease. Long form CASS experience. 1,484 patients with≥ 50% left main coronary artery stenosis initially treated with either surgical or nonsurgical therapy… median survival was NOT prolonged by CABG surgery in patients with normal LV systolic function. Normal LV systolic function defined as 50% or greater. Same with left main equivalent coronary artery disease.

Reimbursement for CABG is $150,000 to 200,000. The motivation is money. The patient be damned. There is a good documentary called "Widomaker" that shows how patients and their families get talked into CABG.

Typically the sales pitch is that the doctor with tell the patient and the patient's wife that he has a **"widow maker"** type of coronary artery lesion. That he should go to the operating room or he could suddenly die from his "widomaker" coronary artery lesion. Almost all patients fall for this.

[My dad fell for this trick. At the time, in my 30's, I didn't know enough about diet and atherosclerosis to talk him out of it. I tried to talk him out of it, but my knowledge wasn't solid enough at that time to convince him. He had the surgery, and did okay with it for four years.

Then, while shoveling snow, he had a vertebral artery dissection, which led to a stroke. I think the vertebral artery dissection was because of the CABG related stapling adjacent to the subclavian artery for the LIMA (left internal mammary artery) to the LAD (left anterior descending artery) arterial graft.]

Neil Armstrong, the first man on the moon, died from what I believe was unnecessary CABG surgery, as described in my September 2012 newsletter.

167

During CABG, the patients sometimes have embolization of atherosclerotic plaque or air bubbles to the eyes, the brain, and other body parts.

Reference: Circulation, 2005, Dec 20; 112(25):3833-8. Retinal (eye) and cerebral microembolization during CABG. Retinal microvascular damage was detected in 5 of 9 CABG patients with cardiopulmonary bypass (on the pump), but in none of the off pump patients. Cognitive iimpairment after CABG is called **"Pump head."**

Reference: "Cognitive outcomes three years after coronary artery bypass surgery: relation to diffusion weighted magnetic resonance imaging. Annals of thoracic surgery. (2008). Mar 85(3):872-9. Found brain damage in 51% of patients.

Reference: NEJM ((2001), Feb 8; 344(6): 395-402. "Longitudinal assessment of neurocognitive function after coronary artery bypass surgery." Five years after bypass surgery 42% of patients showed decline in mental function of 20% or more.

Reference: Thorac Cardiovasc surg, (1988), 96:326-31. Neuropsychological impairment after CABG has been reported in 14-80% of patients, and as high as 100% in the elderly. Why? Because CABG may trigger a stroke. Micro emboli result I cerebral emboli due to toxic chemicals, flakes of plastic equipment, air bubbles, clumps of fat.

Medication therapy of coronary artery disease provides only a small benefit. Primary prevention is treatment of patients with no known heart disease. Secondary prevention is treatment of patients with known heart disease.

The benefit of antiplatelet medications and statins is weak. Most patients can get their total cholesterol below 150 mg/dl (4 IU), with diet, but I sometimes prescribe statins in the ones who need help to achieve that. I sometimes prescribe a baby aspirin daily. I encourage them to exercise without causing chest pain.

The best treatment for coronary artery disease, and the only treatment that works well, is the **low fat, starch based vegan diet with no oil, no avocados, and no nuts or seeds.** With a high fat meal, the oxygen in the blood is reduced by 20%. High fat meal causing decreased delivery of oxygen has been studied by Roy Swank MD, Phd, Peter Kuo MD, Meyer Friedman MD, and Ray Rosenman MD, as well as others.

Reference: M Friedman, Circulation, 29:874, (1964). **Serum lipids and conjunctival circulation after fat ingestion** in men exhibiting type A behavior pattern. Meyer Friedman and Ray Rosenman evaluated blood flow in the eye 4 hours after a 67% fat meal (2 eggs, 4 strips of bacon, milk, cream, bread with 2 pats of butter). They looked at the eye with an 80x magnification. They microscope. They could see small arteries transiently occluding from the blood sludge.

Reference: **Effect of unsaturated fats upon lipemia and conjunctival circulation.** JAMA

Sept (1965) Meyer Friedman Mdand Ray Rosenman MD.

Reference: The **effect of lipemia upon coronary and peripheral arterial circulation** in patients with essential hyperlipemia. Peter Kuo, Am J med (26), Jan 1964.

Reference: Angina pectoris induced by fat ingestion in patients with coronary artery disease. Peter Kuo MD. Jama, July (1955).

Reference: Intravascular aggregation and adhesiveness of blood elements associated with alimentary lipemia… effect on blood brain barrier. Roy Swank. Circulation (9) 1954.

Reference: Effects of stress management training and dietary changes in treating ischemic heart disease. Book: Dr Dean Ornish's program for reversing heart disease. The only system scientifically proven to reverse heart disease without drugs or surgery. In 24 days, a 91% mean reduction in frequency of anginal episodes. In the experimental group, the reported frequency of angina episodes per week decreased from 10.1 before to 1.6 after intervention. Jama (1983) Jan 7;249(1)54-9. and Dean Ornish MD followup article, Am J cardiol 2002, Aug, 90(3), 271-98.

Refrence: Book: Prevent and reverse heart disease by Caldwell Esselstyn MD. Journal of family practice, July 2014. A way to prevent CAD? Vol 63. Articles available at Dr Esselstyn dot com.

Reversal of coronary artery disease has been shown by the work of Walter Kempner MD. EKG's can show cardiac ischemia. Kempner showed many patients who reversed their EKG findings. The work of Nathan Pritikin, as well as Dr's David Blankenhorn, Dean Ornish, and Caldwell Esselstyn has shown that coronary atherosclerosis can be reversed by a low fat, plant based diet.

Atherosclerosis has been around for a long time. Aterhosclerosis occurred in the ancient mummies as shown by lesions in their hearts and aortas. It occurred in European aristocrats who ate diets rich in meats and cheeses. It occurred in the **Alaskan eskimos** who have been eating something similar to the Atkins diet for at least 500 years, and they have a lot of atherosclerosis and osteoporosis. The Eskimos are not healthy. There is no Eskimo paradox.

Reference: Am j clin nutr, 27:916-925, 1974, Bone mineral content of north Alaskan Eskimos by Warren Mather.

The Atkins diet can get a person to lose weight, but it makes them sick. Even his own dat shows that over 70% of the patients are constipated. And they often have bad breath.

As atherosclerotic plaques get older, they often calcify. These calcifications can be seen on a CAT scan of the heart. Calcification is the end stage of inflammation anywhere in the body. When a person has inflmmation elsewhere in the body, the immune system typically heals it, and then a scar is often left over, with a calcification.

I actually had a CAT scan of my chest. I had some coronary artery calcifications. [Likely from his younger years when he ate the SAD diet and smoked cigarettes.] But those are just old scars, they don't do anything. I do not have any angina. I just eat the proper diet, and don't bother with those coronary artery calcifications. - from **Heart disease, truth and treatment** from Dr McDougall you tube channel.

"There are whole populations who before WW2 did not have heart disease. If a whole population could avoid heart disease, then it's unlikely a person has a "genetic" problem that'g going to make them get heart disease…. When a person has **atrial fibrillation,** their cardiac function is decreased by about 25%. The CHADS score is used to determine whether an Afib patient needs anticoagulation." - Dr McDougall.

Dr McDougall newsletter, October 2007, How to keep your arteries clean and reverse atherosclerosis.

All stretched out, humans have 60,000 miles of blood vessels. Your diet effects every inch of these blood vessels. Changing to a plant based, starch based diet helps to improve blood flow. Over months, actual healing of the artery disease (reversal of atherosclerosis) can be demonstrated in almost all patients who follow a low fat, starch based diet.

Dr McDougall, newsletter April 2013, Does olive oil and eating nuts really prevent heart disease.

Describes multiple papers showing that any benefits of Mediterranean diet are likely in spite of olive oil, and added nuts, not because of them.

Dr McDougall newsletter, November 2009, Nuts come in hard shells for a reason.

Dr McDougall newsletter, April 2014, clearing up the confusion surrounding saturated fat by Travis.

Dr McDougall newsletter, September 2010, Statins fail to save lives.

Dr McDougall newsletter, May 2007, and May 2013, who should take statins.

Dr McDougall newsletter, November 2008, Crestor expands the "indications" for statins – and the public suffers.

Dr McDougall newsletter, September 2009, statin therapy, muscle function, and falls in community dwelling older adults. Statins weaken muscles.

Dr McDougall newsletter, July 2012, fish oils fail to prevent heart disease

Dr McDougall newsletter, January 2007, how long to take plavix and aspirin after a DES (Drug Eluting Stent) for the coronary arteries.

Dr McDougall newsletter, March 2006, plavix fails heart patients, and causes bleeding.

Dr McDougall newsletter, August 2004, don't take plavix and aspirin together.

Dr McDougall newsletter, May 2016, beware of interventional cardiologists (heart surgeons).

Dr McDougall newsletter, January 2003, taming elevated triglycerides, insulin resistance, and syndrome X.

Reference: The higher the blood cholesterol, the higher the risk of myocardial infarction. William E. Connor, Preventive medicine, 1972, March, 1(1): 49-83.

Chapter 14. **Dementia**

Dr McDougall newsletter March 2010. Copper and iron from meat damage the brain and body.

Persons in the top 5th of copper intake have a 3x increased risk of cognitive impairment. Authors recommend to avoid almost all multivitamins and mineral pills, because they may contain copper and/or iron.

Avoid eating all meats, because they tend to be plentiful in copper and iron. Copper and iron are much more bio-available from meat, than from vegetable foods. Liver and shellfish are especially high in copper. Red meat is especially high in bio-available iron.

80% of homes in USA have copper pipes for water. Reverse osmosis filters can remove copper from water. [Reverse osmosis, ion exchange, distillation, acid neutralizer systems, and KDF filters can all remove copper from water. Ceramic filters and carbon filters usually cannot remove copper.]

Other metals in our food and water also can cause cognitive impairment, especially aluminum. The western diet is tied to dementia because of the damage from cholesterol and fat in the diet.

The western diet is like the "Broad street pump," and even though we might not agree on exactly what component of it is the main cause of the chronic diseases, all the evidence points to it. The wise thing to do is to avoid the western diet.

Dr McDougall newsletter, March 2004, a natural cure [treatment] for depression.

Dr McDougall newsletter, August 2004, drugs fail for depression.

Dr McDougall newsletter, September 2010, Parkinson's disease and other diet induced tremors.

Parkinson disease is more common in persons who eat the western diet, including white and black Americans. Rural Africans, Chinese and Japanese who's diets are vegan or quasi vegan have much lower rates of Parkinson's disease. Consumption of milk in midlife is associated with increased risk of Parkinson's.

One probable mechanism is the destruction of the blood brain barrier by excess dietary fat. Once this barrier has become abnormally permeable, then auto-antibodies have increased access to brain parenchyma.

Parkinson's disease is possibly an autoimmune disease. There is possibly an increased incidence of Parkinson's disease in multiple sclerosis patients.

Fish and livestock animals bioaccumulate pesticides by eating high on the food chain. When humans eat these foods, they can bioaccumulate pesticides. These pesticides can potentially cause Parkinson's disease.

The chemical harmane is present in beef, pork, and chicken. When cooked at high temperaturesthere is increased concentration of Harmane; worse is with pan frying or grill barbequing.

A plant based, starch based diet helps the body to detoxify.

Dr McDougall September 2009, newsletter, vegetarians make plenty of essential fats (DHA).

Reference: Sanders, Dha status of vegetarians, prostaglandins leukot essent fatty acids, 2009, aug sep;81(2-3):137-41.

Thomas Sanders concluded "in the absence of convincing evidence for the deleterious effects resuliting from the lack of dha in the diet of vegetarians, it must be concluded that needs for omega 3 fatty acids can be met by dietary ALA (Alpha Linolenic Acid, 18:3, n-3). Dha is naturally found in human breast milk. The human body has no difficulty in converting the plant derived omega 3 ALA into DHA or other omega 3 fatty acids, in the liver, thus supplying our needs, even during gestation and infancy.

Dr McDougall June 2009, newsletter, fish is not brain food.

Dietary intake of fish and omega 3 fatty acids in relationto long term dementia risk by Elizabeth Devore in July 2009 of Am J clini nutr found "moderate consumption of fish and omega 3 pufa's do not appear to be associated with long term dementia risk. People who never ate fish had a similar risk of dementia. Had 5,395 patients.

Fish is not health food. Fish is animal muscle, just like muscles of cows and chickens. Fish is loaded with cholesterol, and chemical contaminants.

The most thorough review ever conducted (48 randomized controlled studies of 36, 913 subjects) of fish and omega 3 fats on health was published in ?April 2009 issue of BMJ and authors reported that long chain and shorter chain omega 3 fats do NOT have a clear effect on total mortality, combined cardiovascular events or cancer.

Dr McDougall newsletter, June 2004, Alzheimer's disease can be safely prevented and treated now.

Alzheimer disease (AD) is characterized by the death of brain cells. The main feature of AD is clumps of protein, called beta amyloid deposits, which are commonly referred to as senile plaques, in the extracellular space.

Microtubules inside of cells can become clumped together to form filamentous snarles known as neurofibrillary tangles.

Worldwide the incidence of AD is more common among people who follow meat and dairy centered diets, than among those who eat a more plant based diet.

Estimates are that in developed countries like the USA, 50% of dementia is due to AD, but in developing countries like Africa and Asia, only 35 of dementia is due to AD.

Multiple studies have shown that people eating a diet higher in fat and saturated fat, and cholesterol have at least double the risk of AD. People with advanced atherosclerosis have a much higher risk of AD.

Aluminum is a recognized neurotoxin, that is more toxic to the brain when a person eats a high cholesterol diet. Aluminum increases inflammation.

Aluminum is found in higher concentrations in the brains of persons with AD, than in those without it. Aluminum is found in the senile plaques of beta amyloid.

When aluminum is added to drinking water (for water "purification" to remove turbidity), the populations tend to have a higher risk of AD.

Absorption of aluminum through the gut wall and the blood brain barrier increases with age.

The aluminum chelator desferrioxamine can reduce the pathological concentrations of aluminum in the brain of AD patients down to normal. Desferrioxamine also removes iron from the body. Desferrioxamine can be used to treat Alzheimer's patients.

Aluminum I sthe most abundant metal in the earth crust, and the third most abundant element behind oxygen and silicon.

The human body has ZERO need for aluminum.

Tea is very high in aluminum, but most of it is bound to other substances which limits its absorption.

One should not use aluminum cookware for cooking.

One should avoid medications that contain aluminum, like some antacids, and some analgesics and some calcium supplements.

One should avoid spraying on aluminum antiperspirants. One study showed a 60% greater risk of AD with the use of antiperspirants. All antiperspirants contain aluminum chloride which stops the sweating.

For someone with AD, I would administer desferrioxamine, 125 mg intramuscularly twice daily for 5 days per week for months, maybe years, in order to remove aluminum and iron from the body. By the way, desferrioxamine is a low profit drug that cannot be patented and this is the reason that you have not heard about this treatment."

Dr McDougall newsletter, December 2008, Atkins diet is associated with brain impairment.

Reference: Low carbohydrate weight loss diets. Effects on cognition and mood by Kristen D'Anci in feb 2009 issue of the journal Appetite concluded "present data show memory impairments during low carb diets at a point when available glycogen sotres would be at their lowest. With complete withdrawal of dietary carbohydrate, dieters performed worse on memory based tasks.

"Foods are the most common causes of headache… foods like milk, dairy, eggs, chocolate, corn, wheat, EtOH, tomato, strawberry." - John McDougall MD.

Dr McDougall newsletter, September 2010, better moods from a vegetarian diet

Dr McDougall newsletters on antacids = they are associated with increased risk of dementia, hip fractures, pneumonia (Novermber 2004), and lowering vitamin B12 (March 2008).

Dr McDougall newsletter, March 2012, gum (periodontal) disease and diet.

Chapter 15. **Osteoporosis and Kidneys**

"The main cause of osteoporosis is that people eat too much animal protein; animal protein is acidic. The bones are the main buffer system for dietary acid.

The kidneys excrete the acid protons, and simultaneously excrete calcium. Increased calcium in the urine is called "calciuria." The person is basically peeing their bones into the toilet.

Some of these osteoporosis foundations are just extensions of industry. They promote measurement of bone mineral density (BMD) as a way to sell the osteoporosis drugs.

The funding to get BMD used as a way to determine fracture risk and make recommendations for prescribing medications, was funded by 3 pharmaceutical companies; and the "normal" BMD was based on young women [of around 30 years of age].

Makers of machines to measure BMD, have also sponsored some of the promotional research on using BMD.

This is medically incorrect, because a 30 year old woman carries around more bone density than a postmenopausal woman. The 30 year old woman has that extra bone density so it is available to potentially give her future baby(s).

There's no need for a postmenopausal woman to carry around that extra bone density.
Reference: BMJ 2002, 124, 886-891.

If one uses the "normal" standard as the bones of a 30 year old woman, that makes most women "sick." In women over 50 years old, it leads to 30% of them as being diagnosed with osteoporosis. In women over 65 years old, it leads to 70% of them as being described as having osteoporosis. I do not think that women should undergo BMD testing. There's a 2/3 chance that they will be labeled as "sick"; and there's little chance of benefit, but there's real risk of harm.

Normal bone mass is to be within 1 standard deviation of a 30 yo woman.

Osteopenia is to be within 1 to 2.5 standard deviations of a 30 yo woman.

Osteoporosis is defined as being 2.5 standard deviations below bone mass of a 30 yo woman.

If the woman is > 2.5 standard deviations below the 30 yo woman, and she has a fracture, then she is labeled as having **severe osteoporosis.**

There are many who recognize that BMD is over rated. Eg. the office of health technology

177

assessment of university of British Columbia wrote that "Research evidence does not support either whole population or selective bone mineral density testing of well women at or near menopause, as a means to predict future fractures."

Here's another paper that recommends against BMD screening. "We do not recommend a program of screening menopausal women for osteoporosis by measuring bone density." Included analysis of 11 separate populations and over 2,000 fractures, and found that BMD "cannot identify individuals who will have a fracture." Reference: BMJ, 1996, 312, 1254-1259.

[The BMD can be viewed as a con; the patient is the "mark" or the "chump." The BMD test is the "setup," and the selling of the drug = the payoff."

Bones are the primary calcium buffering system of the body.

The kidneys excrete excess nitrogen. Low protein diets reduce the kidney workload, and protect the kidney. Kempner showed this a long time ago.

Reference: Dr McDougall newsletter, June 2007, save your kidneys, part 2, diet and kidney health.

Animal foods tend to be much more acidic than plant foods. Animal foods have more protein than plant foods. Protein is made out of amino ACIDS. Animal protein has more sulfur containing amino acids like cysteine & methionine. Some of this sulfur gets metabolized into sulfuric acid. This puts an acid load on the body.

The kidneys excrete acid protons = H+ simultaneously with excreting calcium ions. When kidneys are excreting more calcium, that's called calciuria. The calciuria leads to increased risk of calcium stones. Over 95% of kidney stones contain calcium.

PRAL is the Potential Renal Acid Load of a food.

Here is a comparison list of the acid load of various foods = renal acid load per 100 calories of a given food. Notice how much higher the numbers are for animal foods:

Whole milk and low fat milk .2

Egg 5.6 (yolk 7)

Beef 6.3

Chicken 7

Fish (cod) 9.3

Cheddar cheese 10

Fish (salmon) 11

Ground beef 12.5

Mozzarella cheese 16

Swiss cheese 21

Parmesan cheese 34

Now look at the plants where most have negative numbers = are ALKALINE!:

Pasta 7

Roasted mixed nuts 5

Granola bar 4.8

Peanut butter 3.2

Whole wheat bread 2

Peas 1

Wheat flour 1

Beans

White rice .9

Soy milk .6

Instant oatmeal .2

Quinoa -.2

Cucumber -2.5

garlic -3

potato -5

banana -5 → and about the same for cantaloupe & kiwifruit

apples & pears – 5 and about the same for pineapples, blueberries, strawberries, raspberries, peaches

carrots -6

sweet potato -8

baked potatos - 9

Kale -11

Raisins -15

Beet greens -17

tomatos -18

Dried apricots -33

spinach -56

[Most of these numbers taken from Dr McDougall's chart. Some of the numbers taken from other charts of PRAL to make the chart more complete. Both charts agreed in the relative amounts, but were slightly different in the relative amounts.]

Key point: Animal foods tends to be VERY ACIDIC. Beans and grains tend to be minimally acidic. Fruits and veggies tend to be quite ALKALINE, and some starches like potatos are moderately alkaline.

Oxalates in food tend to be bound. If a person eats a low fat diet, the oxalates tend to stay bound to the food, and don't get absorbed. If the person eats a high fat diet, then more of the oxalates separate from the food, and get absorbed into the body.

The Eskimos eat a lot of fish. Fish and all other animal foods are quite similar to each other; this means they all tend to have a lot of fat and protein. Eskimos have a lot of osteoporosis.

In **National Geographic magazine** of June 1987, two eskimo women from 500 years ago, were found frozen in a tomb of ice. They had severe osteoporosis, as predicted by the Eskimo diet that is high in animal protein.

Modern, Alaskan Eskimos are known to have a 10-15% bone deficit compared to USA whites. **Reference:** Am j clin nutr, 27;916, (1974).

A women's age, her family history, and here overall health are more accurate than BMD for prediction of fracture risk.

Soy protein, 25 g, was substituted for an equivalent amount of meat protein for 7 weeks each. The isolated soy protein was just as damaging as meat protein to the bones.

Reference: USA department of agriculture with additional support from the North Dakota beef commision. [I'm no fan of soy, but it sounds to me like this study might be biased against soy.]

Soy protein isolate will likely increase the risk of kidney stones; soy protein isolate also increases ILGF-1, so it might increase the risk of cancer.

Soy protein is a common ingredient in processed foods. For example, eating soy protein bars will increase ILGF-1, and will lead to more calcium in the urine.

That's one of the major pitfalls of animal protein and soy protein. ILGF- increases bone mass. But meat and soy protein isolate also create a big acid load on the body, which may lead to increased risk of cancer. ILGF tends to accelerate the growth of cancer.

Isolated soy protein causes the body to excreate calcium; ie. appears to increase the risk of osteoporosis.

Foods that increase ILGF-1 are usually also high in acid and high in protein. The net effect of foods that increase ILGF-1 that they usually increase the risk of bone loss, kidney stones, and cancer.

Thomas Addis the kidney researcher also showed this. **Reference:** J clin invest 2006 feb 116(2)288-96. Thomas Addis argued from personal clinical experience that reduction in renal "work" by judicious dietary protein restriction was effective in minimizing further loss of kidney function in patients with chronic kidney insufficiency from a variety of causes...

A low protein diet reduces the progression of their kidney disease and death on average by 33-50%." - Dr McDougall.

Bisphosphonates suppress bone turnover. There are some hazards with fosamax and actonel. They can potentially lead to severe bone, joint, and muscle pain.

They can lead to delayed fracture healing. In the long run, over 7 years, they can potentially lead to more fractures. They can sometimes cause bone necrosis (osteonecrosis). See April 2005 McDougall Newsletter." - Dr John McDougall.

Hip fractures tend to be the worst of the osteoporosis fractures. [Osteoporotic spinal fractures can also be a big problem for patients.}

Hormonal replacement therapy (HRT) is not good for preventing osteoporosis fractures. In order to prevent 1 hip fracture, would need to treat 10,000 patients for 2.8 years.

The best way to prevent osteoporosis is to eat a healthy diet, and to exercise. If one of my patients had an abnormal BMD, I would tell her to delay accepting drug treatment. I would tell her to eat a healthy diet, and to exercise, and then, she can repeat the BMD test in two to threee years.

Cow's milk does not prevent osteoporosis. The purpose of cow's milk is to help the calf to grow quickly. Cow's milk is high in IGF-1 (Insulin like Growth Factor-1).

Hormone replacement therapy has only a small effect on fracture risk reduction in women. Approximately 3,100 women must be treated to lead to 1 less fracture annually. **Reference:** Jama, 2004, 291, 2212-20.

Other problems with dairy include:

Dairy protein decreases bowel peristalsis, and can cause constipation.

Dairy lacks vitamin C.

Dairy is a high calorie, high fat food, and is associated with obesity, diabetes, heart disease, heart attacks, and stroke.

It's highly allergenic.

It's associated with autoimmune diseases like type 1 diabetes, and multiple sclerosis.

Dairy can contain environmental contaminants associated with increased risk of Parkinson's disease, and brain damage.

Dairy is associated with increased risk of some forms of cancer.

Dairy can contain a variety of microbes including E. coli, mad cow, bovine leukemia virus.

The purpose of cows milk is to help a baby cow grow rapidly. Cow's milk is not made for humans.

The only good food for infants is human breast milk.

Reference: **Dr McDougall newsletter, January 2004, formula (bottle) feeding causes infant brain damage.**

Human breast milk has 5% of calories from protein. That's all a baby needs! During the most rapid phase of growth in a human's life, we only need 5% of calories from protein. It's reasonable to expect that at other phases of life, our need for protein is less.

A baby should be breast fed. Some of these baby formulas are toxic. A woman should eat a healthy diet before pregnancy and during pregnancy. The mother's diet is important, because it affects her milk.

Beginning around 6 months, a baby can eat some solid food. A baby should NOT eat a low fat diet. Human breast milk is about 50% fat. After weaned from human breast milk, a baby can eat nuts and seeds if it's okay with the pediatrician.

[it seems to me that Dr McDougall believed that the babies be breast fed for at least 6 months if possible.]

The higher a woman's dietary calcium intake, the higher the risk of fractures. Eg. the western countries with high intakes of calcium, like Denmark, United Kingdom, USA, Norway, Sweden, New Zealand, Finland, also have high rates of fractures.

Excess dietary fluoride causes increased bone mineral density; which is called fluorosis; but these are NOT healthy bones. Fluorosis related bones are brittle; are at increased risk for fracture. Thus fluorosis causes INCREASED DENSITY of bones, but the fluorosis bones are at increased risk for fracture!

[Endemic fluorosis is an important problem in India. In USA, most municipal tap water

183

contains fluoride. Spinal fluorosis can mimic the appearance of ankylosing spondylitis, of DISH (diffuse idiopathic skeletal hyperostosis) and OLF (Ossification of Ligamentum Flavum).

- from **How is milk going to make you blind? & Dr McDougall disputes major medical treatments – osteoporosis and the broken bone busine**ss & breast feeding myths and the hidden dangers in your diet, by Dr McDougall from the Dr McDougall Health & Medical center you tube channel.

Dr McDougall newsletter June 2007, save your kidneys, the hard way with medications, part 1.

Protein in urine of 30 mg/day or higher is the hallmark sign for the beginnings of chronic kidney disease. Over 300 mg/day is considered serious kidney disease. In general the more protein in the urine, the worse the kidney disease.

Some medications claim to be renal protective, but lead to increased risk of dying of heart disease. Overtreatment of hypertension can lead to increased risk of cognitive impairement and of heart disease.

Hypertension, elevated cholesterol, and type 2 diabetes are due to the Western diet. Likewise the health of the heart, kidneys, arteries and rest of the body is dependent on a healthy diet. What is missing in the current treatment of people with kidney disease is diet therapy.

Dr McDougall newsletter, March 2011, the best baby formula.

Breast milk is the best food for babies. If the child must have formula, I recommend hypo-allergenic cow's milk formula.

Dr McDougall newsletter January 2011, McDougall diet for pregancy.

As of January 2011, and the father of three grown children, and the grandfather of 3 grandchildren, I have been advising families about nutrition for a long time. The key point is that pregnancy does not change the human diet.

Obesity leads to Caesarian births.

Preeclampsia is a serious sickness of pregnancy.

Morning sickness protects babies from meat.

Fish and omega 3 fats adversely effect pregnancy.

184

Dr McDougall newsletter, May 2004, Food additives do affect your child's behavior, and October 2007, food additives impair child's behavior.

The effects of a double blind placebo controlled artificial food colorings and benzoate preservative challenge on hyperactivity in a general population of preschool children by Bateman in June 2004 issue of Archives of internal medicine found artificial food colorings and a preservative in the diet of 3 yo children caused hyperactive behavior, which reappeared when the chemicals were introduced for 3 weeks. Authors concluded that all **children likely to benefit if artifical dyes and benzoate were removed from their food.**

Dr McDougall, newsletter, September 2009, cholesterol lowering statins weakens muscles and cause falls.

Statin therapy muscle function and falls risk in community dwelling older adults by D Scott published in QJM monthy journal of association of physicians found that "statin use may exacerbate muscle performance declines and falls risk associated with aging without a concomitant decrease in muscle mass, and this effect may be reversible with cessation." A common side effect of statin therapy is skeletal muscle damage (myopathy), which sometimes includes muscle pain (myalgia) and weakness. Muscel enzymes (creatine kinase) may or may not rise in blood with this damage.

When the muscles of patients on statins were evaluated with electron microscopy, it was found that over 70% had muscle cell damage, even when they had not complaints of pain!

The safest, and least expensive way to lower cholesterol is to eat a low fat, no cholesterol diet like the McDougall diet.

Dr McDougall video on protein: **Sarcopenia** is NOT a problem to be solved by eating more protein. Exercise is a helpful treatment for sarcopenia. Extra dietary protein is harmful to the body, to the kidneys, the bones, and the liver.

No one is deficient in protein! No such thing! The studies that say old people need to eat more protein are industry studies. This is fraud, to sell protein supplements and animal foods. Protein supplements aren't just worthless, they're harmful!" - Dr John McDougall.

Chapter 16. **The McDougall Diet**

"The McDougall diet is about 1-2 g or sodium per day." - Dr McDougall from the "stop eating poison" internet lecture.

Dr McDougall, newsletter, January 2008, For the love of grains.

"In Roman times, Ceres was the goddess of agriculture. The gifts offered to Ceres at festivals were "cereal." Grains were considered the "staff of life," the staples of the diet, necessary foods. The most important grains for the romans were wheat and barley. Expressions like the "greatest thing since sliced bread." To keep the plebians happy with bread and circuses. Cash is called "bread," or "dough."

70-83% of the calories from grains are "starch" = complex carbohydrate. Grains are the seeds of grasses = wheat, barley, rice, corn, rye, barley, triticale (a hybrid between rye and wheat), sorghum and millet.

Amaranth, quinoa, buckwheat are derived from broadleaf plants, not grasses, but they are used much like cereal grains.

Starch is a complex carbohydrate. Starch is a polymer of glucose wrapped in fiber. Fruit sugars are simple sugars = simple carbohydrates, not starch. Simple sugars are not a health food. Simple sugars will rot your teeth. Simple sugars are empty calories. Simple sugars raise triglycerides in the blood. Glucose does NOT get much made into fat, but does get burned for energy.

The most important way that I came to the conclusion that humans are starchivores is from this observation: All, large populations of trim healthy people throughout written history have obtained the bulk of their calories from starch.   There are no exceptions!

Examples of thriving people include Japanese and Chinese in Asia eating rice, sweet potatos, and buckwheat. Incas in South America eating potatos. Mayans and Aztecs in Central America eating corn. And Egyptians in the Middle East eating wheat.   People in the middle east have been eating oats for 11,000 years.

Here are the benefits of eating whole grains. Lowers cholesterol, blood sugar, insulin levels, ILGF-1 levels; reduces risk of thrombosis, of heart attack, of type 2 diabetes, of obesity, of colon cancer; helps prevent constipation, increases good gut bacteria, provides antioxidants.

Chapter 17. **McDougall FAQ's**

Dr McDougall, January 2006 Newsletter on Aging in style.

The longest lived person ever, of authentic record, was a French woman who lived to be 122 years of age. There are about 80,000 living centenarians (people 100 yo or older), and almost all of them NEVER saw a doctor before 90 years of age, so it's obvious that medical intervention did not play a role in their longevity.

Average lifespan of Americans in 2002 was 77 years old. Of Japanese in 2002 was 82 years old. Of all Adventists was 85 yo. Of vegetarian Adventists was 87 yo.

Caloric restriction is a proven method to increase longevity in mammals. By switching from meat, dairy, processed foods and oils to a starch based vegan diet, a person typically eats about 400 to 800 fewer calories per day. This spotaneously happens because starches have low caloric density and are very satisfying for the appetite.

Reference: Am j clin nutr, 1987, Dec; 46(6): 886-92.

Another benefit of a plant based diet is that it is high in antioxidants. Antioxidants are health promoting when come from plants. When isolated and put into supplements, antioxidant chemicals are not helpful, and actually increase the risk of sickness and death.

Animal foods, cows milk, soy protein (like in burgers, protein bars, candy bars and other synthetic foods) cause increased ILGF-1 and this may increase aging, and the risk of cancer.

Reference: Ten years of life. Is it a matter of choice? By Gary Fraser & David Shavlik. JAMA, July 9, 2001, Arch intern med; 161(13). SDA's especially the vegan SDA's live much longer than other Californians.

Dr McDougall newsletter, January 2007, the food industry buys nutrition research

Dr McDougall newsletter July 2015, athletics in the spotlight: low carb vs high carb.

The athletic performance of the Tarahumara and the Kenyans and the Ethiopians provide undeniable evidence that the healthiest diets for human beings are very high in carbohydrates.

The Tarahumara average total cholesterol was 125 mg/dL, and triglycerides were 120 mg/dL.

Reference: Wm E. Connor, Am j clin nutr, 1978, Jul;31(7):1131-42.

Dr McDougall, newsletter, September 2010, Better moods from a vegetarian diet.

Vegetarian diets are associated with healthy mood states: a cross sectional study in Seventh Day Adventists by Bonnie L Beezhold, published in the June 2010 issue of the Nutrition Journal found the vegetarian diet profile does not appear to adversely affect mood despite low intake of long chain omega 3 fatty acids. Vegetarians reported significantly less negative emotion than omnivores.

Dr McDougall, newsletter July 2012, lessons from the past, directions for the future: The WW1 starch solution for Denmark.

During WW1, the British naval blockade causes 400,000 Germans (where they continued to eat diets heavy in meat) to die from 1914 to 1918.

Denmark which remained neutral during this conflict was also affected by the blockade, but they thrived; this was due to the brilliance of the physician-nutritionist Mikkel Hindhede (1862-1945).

Based on his suggestions, the people of Denmark switched from a diet plentiful in meat, to one where the bulk of calories came from starchy grains and vegetables. By feeding grains to the population, more food was available. The principal foods for the Danes were bran bread, barley porridge, potatos, greens, milk, some butter.

During the years of food rationing in Denmark, the population actually became healthier, and the death rate from disease was reduced by 34%.

Similar reductions in disease and mortality were seen in WW1 and WW2 in other populations from diabetes, etc.

Dr McDougall newsletter, April 2007, cured meat hurts the lungs.

Dr McDougall newsletter, November 2004, CT-scans, looking for cancer may cause cancer.

Dr McDougall newsletter, December 2010, sleep apnea; too fat to breathe.

Dr McDougall newsletter, February 2004, a little exercise makes a big difference.

Dr McDougall newsletter, October 2005, folic acid supplements are a health hazard.

Dr McDougall newsletter, March 2010, vitamin D pills are of little or no benefit and some harm. So what to do now?

Dr McDougall newsletter, September 2007, low vitamin D: one sign of sunlight deficiency.

Dr McDougall newsletter, May 2005, sunny days, keeping those clouds away. (benefits of sunlight).

Dr McDougall newsletter, August 2004, [your body] a cesspool of pollutants (persistent organic pollutants).

Dr McDougall newsletter, April 2006, non-stick pots and pans, are they safe? April 2006.

Dr McDougall, newsletter, August 2012, The diet wars: the time for unification is now.

Instead of arguing with each other, vegan doctors should be unified against the "real enemy" which is those recommending and profiting from an animal food based diet.

Proponents of a meat and dairy based diet cause sickness, and the profits are reaped by pharmaceutical companies, medical doctors, hospitals, the beef and dairy industry.

Dr McDougall newsletter, May 2008, should you drink 8 glasses of water daily?

People cannot survive more than a few days without water. Hydration helps prevent kidney stones. Hydration does seem to reduce the incidence of headaches. Hydration improves skin tone.

Better to drink bottled water from a glass container, than from plastic. **Reference:** Goldfarb. Just add water. J am soc nephrol, 2008, June; 19(6):1041-3.

Dr McDougall, newsletter, December 2008, The ancient human diet is starch based.

Starch grains on human teeth reveal early diet in northern Peru by Dolores Piperno in Dec 16, 2008 issue of the proceeding of the national academy of science. They found plant parts o nthe deeth of people who lived in northern Peru as long as 11,200 years ago, and concluded these to be indicators of ancient human diets and agriculture. Some of the grains had been cooked. Starch granules from lima beans, commonbeans, peanuts, nuts, squash, grains, and fruits were identified…. Hunter gatherers took advantage of any dependable sources of food, and plants are more available.

Dr McDougall, August 2007 Newsletter: 1. Sex and aging. 2. antacids cause dementia.

Between 1973 and 1976 when I worked on a sugar plantation on the big island of Hawaii, I saw that the Japanese, Chinese and Filipino patients who ate their traditional plant based diets were always trim and usually in excellent health.

191

The elderly Filipino men would save their money for retirement, and then go marry a 20 year old Filipino woman, and bring her back to Hawaii. Everyday, a family consisting of a seventy year old (plus) gentleman and his 20 yo bride, and their children would come into my medical office. For these men, a diet of rice and vegetables meant a much more interesting life.

Men eating the western diet were not so fortunate. Erectile dysfunction is caused by decreased arterial blood flow to the penis due to atherosclerosis. ED is sometimes reversible by eating a diet of starch and vegetables.

Histamine 2 receptor antagonists like cimetidine (tagamet), ranitidine (zantac) and famotidine (pepcid) are a risk factor for cognitive impairment 2.5x higher risk!

Dr McDougall, newsletter July 2004, Coffee – pleasure or pain.

Coffee increases blood cholesterol both total and LDL cholesterol, and blood triglycerides. On average cholesterol is increased by 10%. This increased cholesterol might cause increased risk of heart attack.

Coffee raises blood pressure. Decaf coffee also increases blood pressure about 2 to 54 mm Hg. Coffee is upsetting to the stomach by reducing function of the lower esophageal sphincter. Allows gastric acid to reflux into the esophagus.

Coffee is associated with increased risk of irregular heart beats (arrhythmias), nervous tremor, headaches, anxiety, teeth grinding, jaw clenching, insomnia, frequent urination, elevated eye pressure (glaucoma), diarrhea, osteoporosis, and periodontal disease.

When quit coffee, may have withdrawal symptoms for 1 week.

Dr McDougall, newsletter December 2012, people should avoid annual physical exams.

The Nordic Cochrane center systematic review found that genral health check did NOT reduce morbidity or mortality, but the number of new diagnoses was increased.

Dr McDougall newsletter, February 2005, Popular diets.

"In the short term, at 1 year followup, most diets will lead to some weight loss, and often reduce several cardiac risk factors. In the long run, it's a different story.

Dean Ornish MD said that his low fat, near vegetarian diet has been scientifically shown to reverse atherosclerosis, decrease angina (chest pain), bring about permanent weight loss (5 years or longer), and reduce cardiac events (such as heart attacks) by 2.5 times. The other diets have no published research that shows benefits for heart disease.

The main reason most diets fail is that people cannot adhere to them long term.

You will notice that the McDougall diet is seldom included in research studies done by others. The McDougall diet is based on the history of human nutrition; of human anatomy and physiology; of human health research.

The McDougall diet is focused primarily on health, rather than weight loss. The weight loss comes with time, and is sustainable.

You never have to be hungry with the McDougall diet. The health benefits are extraordinary. The McDougall diet helps people to have a higher quality of life, and to remain more productive.

The foods recommended in the McDougall diet are very inexpensive. [Starches are cheap.]

People save time and money by avoiding medications, doctors, and hospitals.

Clear rules with distinct boundaries are easier to follow than "moderation," which distinguishes the McDougall diet from other low fat diets.

The McDougall 7 day program:

Followup of 1,703 patients after eating McDougall diet for 7 days with an unrestricted amount of food:

- Average weight loss of 3.1 lbs.

- Average reduction in total cholesterol 22 mg/dl.

- Average decrease in blood pressure (for those whose initial BP was > 140/90) was 18/11 mm Hg.

- Nearly 90% were able to get off blood pressure and diabetic medications.

McDougall diet was also tested at **Oregon Health and Science University** with MS (multiple sclerosis) patients. 85% of them were compliant for 12 months. McDougall diet group ate 12.5% of calories from fat. Control group ate 37.5% of calories from fat. Average weight loss after 12 months was 19 lbs, while eating unrestricted amounts of food. Average reduction in total cholesterol was 19 mg/dl. Patients noted a reduction in fatigue.

McDougall diet also underwent an independent analysis over 12 months in **New Zealand = BROAD study.** One year in a community based setting, in Gisborne, New Zealand, with 65 participants, 35-79 yo.

Average weight loss was 25.3 lbs in one year, while eating an unrestricted amount of food. The patients were not told to exercise (they could if they wanted). Medication usage decreased by 29%. Average total cholesterol reduction was 21 mg/dl.

Reference: The BROAD study: a randomized, controlled trial using a whole food plant based diet in the community for obesity, ischaemic heart disease or diabetes. McHugh. Nutr & diabetes, 7, 256, (2017).

"You can EXPECT these [great] results" – Dr McDougall as he showed numerous patient who lost large amounts of weight, and improved their health.

Carl Lewis, world champion sprinter and long jumper had great success while eating the McDougall diet. **Reference:** Runner's world, August 1992.

"Our body responds to sugar with the output of more energy for exercise" – Dr McDougall.

"If you don't take estrogen replacement therapy, then fibroids disappear after menopause… the western diet tends lead to earlier age onset of puberty in girls, age 12, instead of age 16, and to delay the onset of menopause a few years, to age 52 (instead of age 48 years old), and this increases the risk of fibrocystic breast disease, breast cancer, abnormal uterine bleeding. This prolonged estrogen stimulation wreaks havoc on the female reproductive system… " - Dr McDougall.

"Nathan Pritikin pointed out decades ago that Americans were eating way too much fat. Pritikin said that the best way to classify diets was based on the amount of fat.

Diet are usually high in fat or high in carbohydrates.

The human body has over 60,000 miles of arteries. Atherosclerosis doesn't just occur in the heart. The high fat diets are causing atherosclerosis throughout the arterial system. Pritkin described the problems from a high fat diet as "lipotoxicity."

Blockage of an artery in the heart is a heart attack. Blockage of an artery in the brain is a stroke. Blockage of arteries in the kidneys causes kidney failure. Blockage of the arteries of the penis causes impotence. That's the most common cause of impotence.

Macular degeneration is the most common cause of blindness in adults. Macular degeneration is related to atherosclerosis blockage of arteries in the eye.

Reference: Dr McDougall newsletter, April 2013, Macular degeneration is due to the

Western diet.

Blockage of arteries to the hearing apparatus causes hearing loss.

Blockage of the arteries to the foot causes gangrene, and is often requires treatment with amputation.

Blockage of arteries to the spine causes disc degeneration. Blockage of arteries to the gut causes a bowel infarction.

When you eat a low fat, starch based vegan diet to prevent atherosclerosis of the heart, you are also helping to prevent atherosclerosis every where else in the body." - From Heart disease Truth and Treatment by Dr McDougall at his you tube channel.

The **glycemic index** is quite over rated.   Blood sugar is supposed to go up after you eat. For example, a boiled potato is a very healthy food, and it has a glycemic index of 101. Fructose has a glycemic index of only 20, but it tends to cause fatty liver, and to elevate blood triglycerides.

It's normal, after eating a starch, for your blood glucose to go up to around 140-150.

For a more detailed discussion of glycemic index, please see **Dr McDougall's newsletter from July 2006 called "Glycemic index – not ready for prime time."**

The real question with a treatment is whether it provides a benefit like cures you of a disease or helps you to live longer. Be careful with industry sponsored risk assessments. The important thing is **ABSOLUTE RISK** and not **relative risk.**

Relative risk estimates can greatly exaggerate the "benefits" of a drug. All they have to do is compare the drug to a lousy treatment or placebo, and this can make the drug seem great by comparison.

However, in these same cases, the drug often has very little absolute risk benefit. Eg. something like benefits 1 out of 1,000 for the condition of treatment; but has potential side effects in all of those 1,000 who took the drug."

Eg. Fosamax is proclaimed to have a 50% relative risk reduction for fractures, but the actual absolute risk reduction is only 1.7%; and fosamax has many potential side effects like can't lay down after eat, can cause severe bone pain, delays fracture healing, and at 7 years, one might have increased fracture risk, and can get jaw bone osteonecrosis.

Notice how there's a big difference between the sound of the relative risk, and the absolute risk. Upon hearing the fosamax relative risk reduction of 50%, the average person might think, "I would be foolish not to take Fosamax."

However, upon learning that the absolute risk reduction for fractures is only 1.7%, they are able to make a more informed choice.

- from videos "Eating starches makes my blood sugar spike. How is that good? & **Dr Mcdougal disputes major medical treatments**" by Dr John McDougall at his you tube channel.

Dr McDougall, June 2009, newsletter, real healthcare reform has HEALTH as the primary goal. And May 2012 newsletter, converting to a starch based diet in medical practice.

In 1986, shortly after starting my 12 day live in program at St Helena hospital, I had several meetings with representatives from major medical insurance companies, with the intention of having my treatment, called the McDougall Program paid for by a patient's medical insurance.

I showed that the program would cost $5,000 instead of cardiac bypass surgery at $45,000 (if all went well). I expected a favorable response from the insurance companies.

However, the insurance companies were not interested. They said that my program required the patients to change their diets, and the insurance company didn't believe they would. Open heart surgery does not require any cooperation from the patient, other than to lay down on the operating table.

I pushed my arguments farther, but they still didn't go for it. Then one said, "You don't get it. We take a piece of the pie, and the bigger the pie, the more we get."

In 1978, the day after my graduation from my internal medicine residency at the university of Hawaii, I fold my former boss, that 80% of the disease I care for is caused by the rich Western diet, and most of the sickness can be greatly benefited and/or cured with a change to a starch based diet. The disgruntled look on his face made me think he would have torn up my diploma if he had the chance.

My former boss told me, "John, I like you and your family. But I am concerned that you will starve to death with your crazy ideas about food. All you will collect for patients is a bunch of bums and hippies."

My response was, "So be it. Then I will starve. Because I cannot prescribe drugs and surgeries that I know will do my patient smore harm than good."

More importantly, I think my former boss was really trying to tell me was that I was going to fail financially because I was not playin by the traditional rules set by years of economic pressures for a successful medical practice. The way for general doctors to make a secure living is to collect a bunch of patient sand get them hooked on medications for blood pressure, diabetes, cholesterol, pain, etc.

I departed my former boss's office with these words, "I believe you are wrong. My practice will be made up of successful people who have made great sacrifices to get an education, build businesses, and develop successful relationships…. These people will seek me out, to help improve their health."

History shows that I was right, and he was wrong. I am the luckiest doctor in the world. Not only do I make an adequate income (like most doctors do), but I also have the satisfaction of seeing my patients heal and stay healthy (like most doctors don't).

Sick people take medications. Healthy people don't.

Article then summarizes Dr McDougall's approach to weaning patients off of hypertension and type 2 diabetes medications.

[The insurance companies are in on it. Drug companies, device manufacturers, hospital corporations, and insurance companies all benefit from increasing patient usage of the health care system; from taking the patient's money.]

Dr McDougall newsletter, September 2009, Profound statements from the former editor of JAMA (from 1982-1999), Dr George Lundberg.

Dr Lundberg said, "I believe that there are still many ethical and professional American physicians and many intelligent American patients who are capable of, in an alliance of patients and physicians of doing the right things.

Academic medical centers should take the lead, rather than continuing to teach new doctors to take the money and run."

Then Dr McDougall added, #1. require all doctors and dieticians to teach a starch based diet. #2. Earnestly promote clean habits and exercise. #3. Make baby formula by prescription only. #4. Outlaw the sale of all oral diabetic medications. #5. Treat elevated blood pressure only if sustained for months at over 160/100 mm Hg. Use chlorthalidone to lower it only down to 140/90."

Chapter 18. **The Potato**

"If I was only allowed to eat one food, I would choose the potato.

If I had to pick one food to save humanity, it would be the potato.

Potatos have the highest calorie yield per unit of farmland, compared to any other crop.

The potatos grows under ground, and is a complete food. It has all the nutrients except for vitamin B12.

People have called me, Dr Potato, and I like that.

Potatos provide ideal nutrition; not just adequate nutrition, but ideal nutrition.

Boiling and baking are good ways to cook potatos.

Potatos have only 1% of calories from fat. Populations who eat a lot of potatos are trim and health. For example, in Peru, where they eat a lot of potatos, they are trim and healthy.

[Potatos have a lot more potassium than sodium. One serving of plain potatos has 379 mg of potassium, and 4 mg of sodium. That's a K factor ratio of potassium:sodium of 95:1. To prevent hypertension, it's recommended by Richard Moore MD, Phd to eat at least a K factor of 5:1. Dr Rogers believes K factor of around 10:1 or more is better.]

Sweet potatos are very much like potatos. In Papua New Guinea where they used to get 92% of their calories from sweet potatos, they were trim and healthy.

To be healthy you just need: clean water and air. Moderate activity (exercise). Sunshine. Comfortable surroundings. Companionship. Plant based, starch based diet. Returning to your religious roots can also help to lower stress.

Potatos are an excellent food for athletes. Potato puree (mashed potatos) can serve as a race feeding strategy to support prolonged exercise performance for trained cyclists, maintaining blood glucose concentration, facilitating gastric emptying, and supporting cycling performance. (Comparable to commercial CHO gel products). Potatos are a cost effective, whole food, nutrient dense, source of CHO.

Potatos have been called the anti-scurvy vegetable. Potatos are very cheap. Potatos went from South America, (they originated in the Andes), to Europe in the 1600's. Potatos provided abundant food; this extra food availability enabled an increase in population for England and Wales in the 1800's.

Potatos can grow to maturity in as little as 50 days. One acre of potatos can feed 10 people for a year. When stored under cool, dry, well vented conditions, potatos can be stored for years.

Infants can do well when fed potatos. **Reference:** J nutr 1981; Oct; 111(10):1766-71.

In world war 1, the Danes switched from eating animal foods, to eating potatos, and they did very well during the time of rationing. The Germans continued to eat large amounts of animal foods, and hundreds of thousands starved to death.

In 1925, a 25 year old man, and a 28 year old woman, under close medical supervision, ate a diet of almost entirely potatos, and they came out of it as healthy as ever. **Reference:** Biochemical J, 1928, 22;22:258-260.

Charles Voight, the director of the his state's potato commission ate 20 potatos a day for 60 days straight. He lost 21 lbs while eating 2,200 calories of potatos per day. His total cholesterol went down 67 points. **Reference:** 20 potatoes a day dot com.

Andrew Taylor went on a potato diet, and lost 117 lbs in one year. He has online videos. He wrote a book called "Spud fit."

If you are sick, and you don't know what to do, and you are too distracted at the moment to study and think in more detail: then just eat potatos! Potatos are superior nutrition.

Potatos is one of the best foods, if not the best food for satisfying hunger.

Healthy foods are way cheaper than hospital bills.

Potatos and sweet potatos are almost the same. Sweet potatos and yams are almost the same.

Potatos are as good as rice for lowering blood sugar in type 2 diabetes. **Reference:** Am j clin nutr, 1984, Apr, 39(4): 598-606.

Potatos grow most efficiently at the Northern latitudes like in Idaho and Wisconsin of the USA. One can grow more potatos per acre than any other starch. Potatos are drought tolerant. Potatos are also heat tolerant. Potatos are disease resistant.

It takes 4x as much land to grow the equivalent amount of rice as potatos. It takes about 6x as much land to grow the equivalent amount of wheat as potatos.

Potatos, as a crop, produce the most food energy per liter of water used on the plant.

In the future, the world would be better off if we ate more potatos. I think we're going to have to eat more potatos and rice.

Do not eat the spud roots of potatos because they can contain increased amounts of solanine. When potatos spoil, they can accumulate a toxic chemical called solanine. Solanine is especially in the green stuff on spoiled potatos, and in the spud roots; do not eat these. Throw out the spoiled potatos. Potatos are cheap.

Side effects of eating solanine can include headache, diarrhea, nausea, vomiting, weakness, depression, and finally paralysis. A rare skin disease called "potato eruption."

Death from solanine poisoning is rare.

[I've eaten potatos every week for many decades, and have never had a problem from eating potatos. If a potato looks spoiled, eg. has green discoloration, I throw it out. If it has spud roots, ("grows eyes"), then I break them off, and throw them away.

- from **Potato mastermind parts 1 & 2** by Dr McDougall at Dr McDougall Health & Medical Center you tube channel.

Chapter 19. **Dr Mcdougall quotes**

"Some of the other famous nutrition experts are jealous of Dr McDougall, because he's the best expert." - anonymous.

The ADA diet is designed to make sure the diabetes patient is never cured – Nathan Pritikin.

Dr McDougall Quotes:

"In the 1970's, the plant based manual laborers in Hawaii would retire at 65; go to the Philipines to get a new young wife; have a new family with no viagra; live healthy into their late 80's.

The nutrition journals were more reliable before the mid 1980's when many were bought by big companies.

It is absolutely essential to get some sunshine… vitamin D in a pill form is toxic; they can lead to increased risk of falls and fractures …

Dr. Kempner is one of my heroes… Ancel Keys was a good man who did good research… Denis Burkitt was the first one to tell me that diet had anything to do with disease...

hard cheeses are the most acidic foods…

Populations eating meat, oil, junk food is just a blip in history in the last 50-100 years… before that, only kings and queens ate a lot of meat…

In the long ago days, before tobacco, and air pollution and processed food, the Kings and Queens of the past who ate a lot of meat had atherosclerosis related disease.

I'm the luckiest doctor in the world, because my patients get better…

You're not gonna win in the medical business. The smart option is to get out of the medical business, safely. You get out of the medical business by becoming healthy. Eat a healthy diet. Exercise. Get off medication.

I've seen three generations raised as vegans. They're healthy and they're smart.

What keeps me going isn't fame or fortune, it's my patients. The real reward comes from sitting down with one person and making a difference in their life….

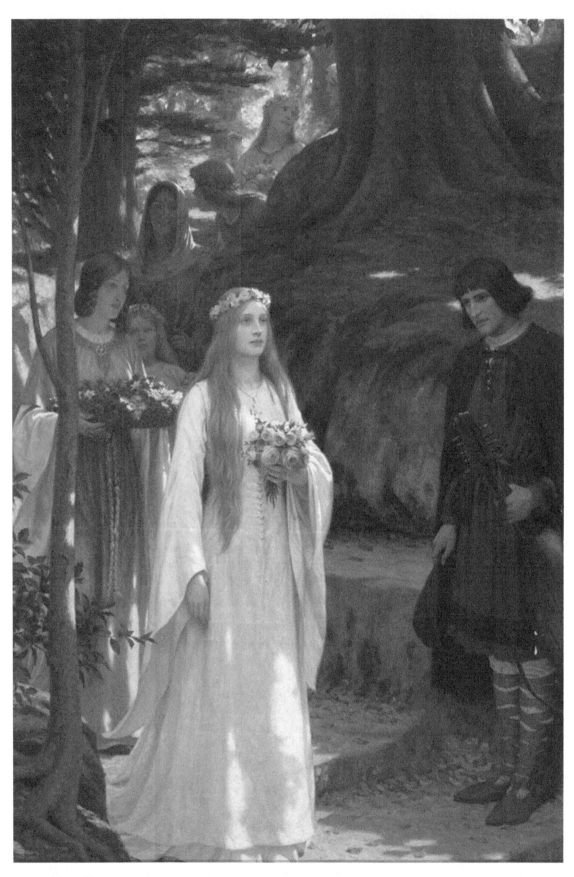

Fig 19-1: **My Fair Lady** by Edmund Leighton, 1914, public domain. Working together in the operating room, **John Mcdougall meets Mary,** and it's LOVE AT FIRST SITE.

Starch has unlocked the door to good health for thousands of my patients...Starch is better than fruits for satisfying hunger.

There's no such thing as a fruitarian population..

The gladiators were barley men.

Sweet potatos are probably the healthiest food...

Starch is a better name than complex carbohydrate. Complex carbohydrate confuses people…

Starch is what the human body needs. Starch is what satisfies hunger. All large healthy populations eat a starch based diet. There are no exceptions…

Eating starch is the most important thing for health. Starch is cheap. "Humans are starchivores." Most of your calories – about 90% - should come from COOKED STARCH.

STARCH is the SOLUTION to how to become HEALTHY!

You can see the truth. Starch eaters are thin and healthy… Before 1970 when the Chinese at 90% of their calories from rice, a billion out of a billion were thin...

If you want to help someone to become healthier, teach them how to eat a low fat, starch based, whole food, plant based diet.

The McDougall diet is a cost free, side effect free treatment for most of the chronic western diseases.

Kempner showed plant based dietary reversal of coronary artery disease by EKG in the 1940's;

Pritikin showed it in the 1960's.

Blankenthorn showed it by cardiac cath in the 1970's;

Ornish showed it in the 1990's.

The ability to partially reverse coronary artery disease with a plant based diet has been known for a long time.

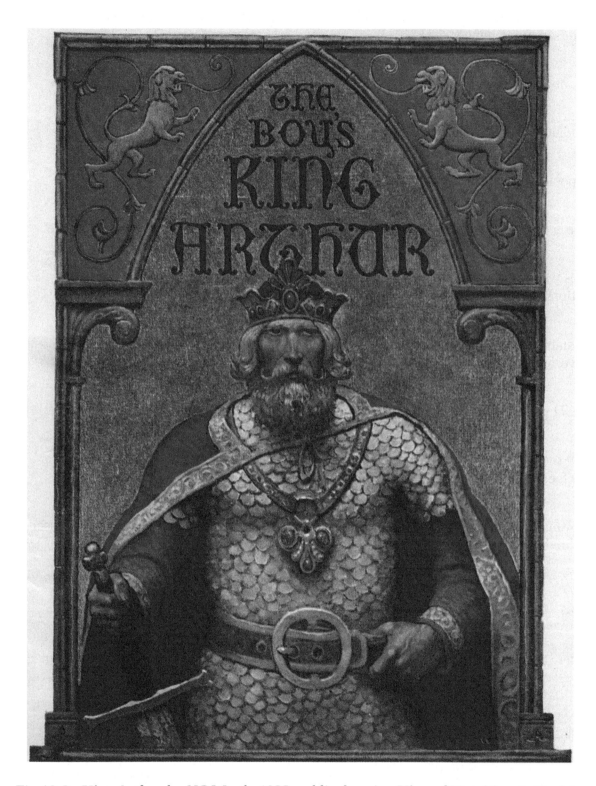

Fig 19-2: **King Arthur** by NC Wyeth, 1922, public domain. **King of Nutrition & Health, John McDougall MD.**

People can NOT cut down on a food. They have to stop eating it. They have to stop eating animal foods and oils.

It's just like alcohol and cigarettes. They can't cut down. They have to stop those things.

In all my years as a doctor [45 years], I've never seen a smoker or an alcoholic be successful "cutting down." They must quit 100%.

There is no such thing as a dietary deficiency of omega 3 fat from a plant based diet… essential fat deficiency is essentially unknown in free living populations…

Blankenthorn's data showed that only TOTAL reduction of dietary fat was beneficial for reduction of atherosclerosis.

Change in type of fat did not provide a significant benefit.

Fat paralyzes the insulin receptor. J Shirley Sweeney's experiment indicated this back in the 1920's. A high fat meal was fed to medical students and their sugars went up.

Type 2 diabetes is 100% curable… It's pretty much impossible to get type 2 diabetes while eating the McDougall diet… The McDougall diet is a low fat, starch based, vegan diet…

Nuts have 80-95% fat and should be kept to a minimum.

Fat makes cancer grow. Sugar does not.

High fat meal decreases PO2 by 20%… Waarburg said that he could turn normal cells into cancer cells by depriving them of oxygen.

No naturally occurring diet could be too low in protein or calcium… There has never been a report of dietary calcium deficiency… I've never seen a case of protein or calcium deficiency…

there is no such thing as a dietary protein deficiency from a naturally chosen diet…

Old people don't need more protein. Old people need to eat less food. It's normal for old people to be thinner… people get sick when protein gets 35% or higher; it's called "rabbit starvation."

You should be suspicious of conventional doctors. You should view them as businessmen; like used car salesmen… the average doctor knows no more about nutrition than his secretary, unless she's on a diet, then she knows more…

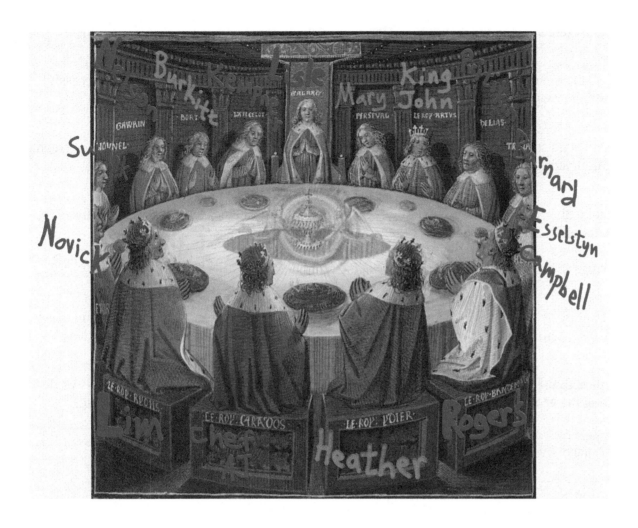

Fig 19-3: **King Arthur and the Round Table of Knights with a vision of the Holy Grail i**n the center of the table by Edvard d'Espinques, 1475, public domain. King John McDougall and Queen Mary and Princess Heather with their students.

The Heimlich maneuver works, but the back slaps do not. Heimlich maneuver pushes air upward, and helps to clear the airway of an ingested foreign body… back slaps can cause the foreign body to become more deeply lodged in the airway.

For near drowning patients, the first step is to get the water out of the lungs… the Heimlich maneuver helps to get the water out of the lungs.

It's better to be hated, than ignored, when change is the goal… To reduce healthcare costs, all doctors and dieticians should be required to teach a starch based diet…

Industry food seeks unique positioning: meat with protein; dairy with calcium; fish with omega 3 fats…

Just say "no" to animal foods and oils. Oil is added to food because it gets the salt and sugar to stick to the food...

Baby formula should be by prescription only…

all oral diabetic medications should be outlawed, ..

Hypertension should only be treated with medications after it has been sustained for months at 160/100 mm Hg or higher. The best medication for HTN is the diuretic, Chlorthalidone. BP should be lowered to no less than 140/90 with medication...

Do not take supplements; the only exception is vitamin B12… the only valid criticism of the vegan diet is the need to supplement with vitamin B12...

The best way to determine water intake is to go by thirst...

They try to block me, and I run around them….

Aluminum spray deodorants are worse than roll ons, because people inhale the aluminum, and it can go along the olfactory system to the brain...

You can live on only potatos and a vitamin B12…Potatos have the highest yield per acre of any starch… Potatos are the working man's food. Potatos are cheap. Potatos make people healthy. The potato pulp has about the same nutrition as the potato skin…

The claim that our ancestors needed meat to develop a big brain is not true.

If we eat natural plant foods, we will always, during all stages of life, get enough omega 3 fats.

Since the beginning of humans on earth, most populations were land bound, and did not eat fish… for humans, our need for fat is very minimal...

Happiness comes from helping other people…

Patients with rheumatoid arthritis or psoriasis often show improvement within one week,

and markedly decreased pain by 4 months when they become vegans.

Coffee is not a health food. It's best to avoid it…

People love to hear "good things" about their bad habits...

The Atkins diet is the make yourself sick diet… the Kempner diet is the diet for the nearly dead… **the McDougall diet is for the living**…

The most common reason people fail when they try to eat a vegan diet is because they don't eat enough starch, or because they continue to eat oils…

"Most chronic disease is not a mystery. It is caused by eating the wrong food."Fix the food, and you fix 80% of medical problems…. To cure chronic disease, the key is to stop sources of repeated injury [animal foods and oils]… In order to get the cure, you must stop the cause…

The key to longevity is to increase carbohydrate intake, and to decrease intake of protein and fat… you want to lower your ILGF… increased ILGF makes you look older, and die sooner...

Dairy, meat and oil cause leaky gut and autoimmune arthritis.. Vegetable oil is toxic to the intestinal lining.

There are no benefits to eating vegetable oil or fish oil.

Vegetable oils are powerful tumor promoters.

Chinese and Japanese women in the 1970's who ate a rice based diet had almost no breast cancer…

I've never seen a single case of arsenic poisoning from rice, or for any other reason...

People who try to satisfy hunger with vegetables fail, and they sometimes go back to eating meat…

Animal foods and oils are poisons.

Meat is animal muscle. Animal muscle is pretty much the same in all animals [mammals]...

Meat is a poison. All animal foods are bad. They're all high animal protein, high fat [except skim milk] and low fiber...

Foods are the most common causes of headache... foods like milk, dairy, eggs, chocolate, corn, wheat, EtOH, tomato, strawberry.

People who lie and say keto diet is good, are evil... The Keto paleo diet is dangerous and dishonest... There are multiple studies that show that low carb diets are associated with an increase in cardiovascular disease, and all cause mortality; there are no studies that show the opposite...

the people who promote paleo, keto, low carb diets are liars... the goal of the low carb movement is to hide the truth...

Writing the newsletter is the only thing that has kept me learning. It usually takes me about 1-2 weeks to write each one, and I write it once a month...

Human breast milk has only 5% of calories from protein; and that is the most rapid phase of growth of our lives. Breast milk is ideal. It hast to be, or babies would not survive. Adults are not growing like that. Adults do not need that much protein. Adults likely only need about 3% of their calories from protein...

Hunter gatherers were mostly gatherers...

You don't nd to eat a wide variety of foods.

Smoothies are over rated; you don't make a food healthier by hitting it with a blade 1,000 times...

Kempner was able to show retinal photographs of diabetic retinopathy reversal. We can see the eyes. Something similar to that is happening all throughout the body...

When people lose weight, they transiently get increased blood cholesterol as the cholesterol moves out of their fat cells, and their fat cells shrink...

Dairy companies say that chocolate milk is "nutrition in disguise." I say it's disease in disguise."...

The Western diet is food poisoning, and it causes acne, constipation, GERD, obesity, hypertension, diabetes, coronary artery disease, arthritis… my food poisoning book is available on my website for free (Dr McDougall dot com). The main causes of food poisoning are animal foods, and free oils.

If something is right, it should be right, however you look at it, because it's true.

Statins should only be given to people with high risk of heart disease, and not to anyone with elevated cholesterol numbers.

The best diet for diabetics is a low fat, starch based, vegan diet with no oils…

Why manage type 2 diabetes with pills, when you can CURE IT with diet?"

- John McDougall MD.

"When you feed herbivores a high fat diet, they all get atherosclerosis… elevated blood cholesterol is the main risk factor for coronary artery disease" – William Roberts MD, best cardiac pathologist in the world.

"Elevated LDL cholesterol sticks red blood cells together. This is called "overcoming the zeta potential." This increases blood viscosity. Makes the blood thick. Thick blood causes hypertension, and atherosclerosis." - Gregory Sloop MD, pioneer of atherothrombosis theory, and best atherosclerosis expert in the world.

"Fiber is life, pharma is death" – Jeff Wilson, nutrition expert, runs YT channel, Veg Source, and VegSource.com.

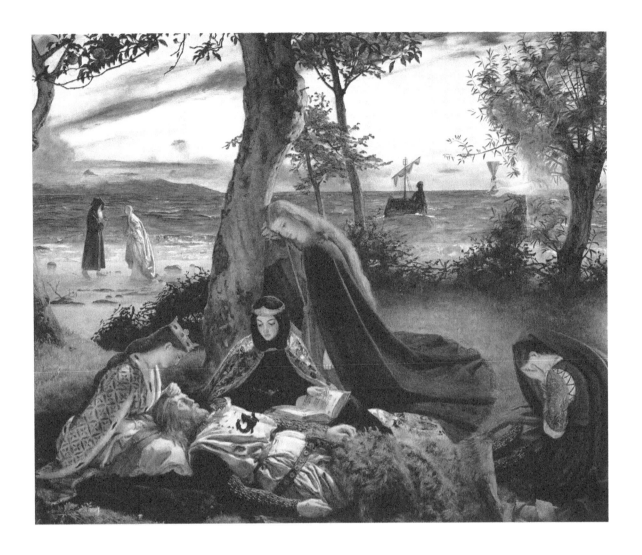

Fig 19-4: The death of King Arthur by James Archer, 1860, public domain.

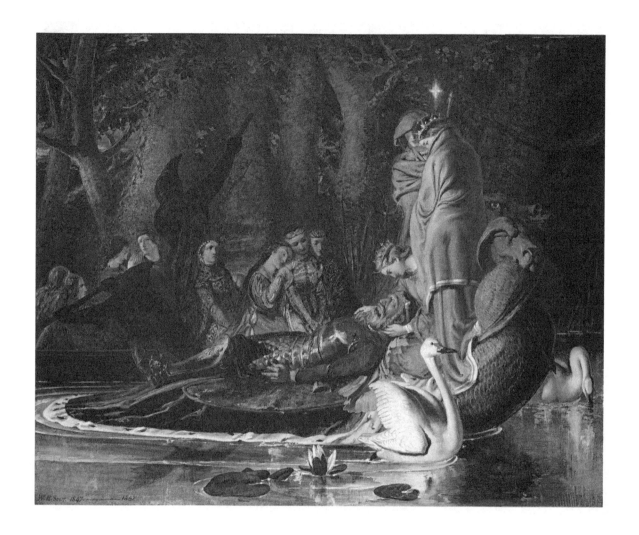

Fig 19-5: **The death of King Arthur** by Wm Bell Scott, 1862, public domain.

"Yet some men say

in many parts of England

that King Arthur is not dead...

and that he shall come again,

and he shall win the Holy Cross."

                    - Thomas Mallory.

Chapter 20. **References**

These references are useful for debates about common nutrition topics.

Kempner stuff

Scientific publications of Walter Kempner MD, volume 2. Available at Dr McDougall dot com.

"Otto Warburg: cell physiologist, biochemist, eccentric" by Hans Krebs, copyright 1981, (definitive biography of Warburg).   Krebs was his student.

"Fat like us" book by Jean Renfro Anspaugh, copyright 2001.

"Secrets of ultimate weight loss" book by Chef AJ, copyright 2018.

Kuo (1955) "**Angina pectoris induced by fat ingestion** in patients with coronary artery disease" JAMA 158: 1008-13.

Friedman (1965) "**Effect of unsaturated fats upon lipemia & conjunctival circulation**" JAMA 193: 882-86

Swank (1961) "Biochemical basis of MS" Springfield IL, Charles Thomas pub.

Winitz (1970) "Studies in metaboloic nutrition employing **chemically defined diets**" Amer J clin nutr 23: 525-45

McKean (1970) "Grow of phenylketonuric children on **chemically defined diets**" Lancet I:148

Kempner (1975) "Tx of massive obesity with rice reduction diet program." Analysis of 106 pts with at least 45 kg wt loss" arch int med, 135: 1575-1584.   avg wt loss 64 kg = 141 lbs. Also found on p. 516 of 570 in Kempner's "Scientific publications, vol 2."

 Blankenhorn (1978) "Rate of atherosclerosis change during Tx of hyperlipoproteinemia" circ 57:355-61.

 Astrup (1973) "CO, smoking, & CV dz" circ 48: 1167-68. Lowering blood oxygen only 15-20% caused increased endothelial permeability & subintimal edema.

Sweeney (1927) "Dietary factors influence dextrose tolerance test" Arch int med, 40: 818-30.

Goldblatt (1953) "**Induced malignancy in rat subjected to anaerobiosis**" j exp med 97:525-52.

Warburg "Prime cause and prevention of cancer" editor Dean Burk, **35% reduction of O2 was able to induce cancer**.

Hypertension stuff:

215

Bassett (2003) "How much exercise is required to reduce blood pressure in essential hypertensives?" Am J HTN, August, 16 (8):629-633

Madias (2007) "Sodium & potassium in pathogenesis of HTN" nejm, May 10;356 (19): 1966-78

Madias (2014) "Impact Na+ & K+ on HTN risk" semin nephrol, 34:257

McCullough (1997) "Aging, salt intake, and HTN in Kuna of Panama" HTN, Jan;29 (1 pt 2): 171-6

Jurgens (2012) "Effects of low Na+ diet vs high Na+ diet on BP, renin, aldosterone, catecholamines, cholesterol, and triglyceride" Cochrane review. Am J HTN, Jan; 25 (1) : 1-15.

Williams (1957) "Increased blood cell agglutination following ingestion of fat, a factor contributing to cardiac ischemia, and anginal pain" Angiology 8:29-39

Donnison (1929) "BP in African native" Lancet, 213 (5497) : 6-7.

Beegom (1997) "Higher saturated fat with higher risk HTN in urban population south India" int j cardiol, 58:63-70

Oliver (1975) "BP, sodium intake in Yanomamo" Circulation, 52 (1): 146-51.

Gleibermann (1973) "BP & dietary salt in human populations" ecol food nutr, 2:143-56. Linear relat betw salt intake & BP.

Matrai (1986) "Blood rheology in vegetarians" br j nutr, 56: 555-60.

Kempner (1949) "Treatment of heart, kidney & hypertensive disease with rice diet" ann int med, 31 (5): 821-56

"Pritikin Program for diet & exercise" book by Nathan Pritikin, copyright 1979.

"Starch solution" book by John McDougall MD, copyright 2012.

"How not to die" book by Michael Greger MD, copyright 2013.

Wenner (2013) "High dietary sodium impairs endothelium" J Htn, 31 (3):530-6.

Barrett (2014) "Postprandial effect high salt meal on arterial stiffness, nitric oxide" atherosclerosis, 232 (1): 211-6.

Ref: Swank stuff.

RL Swank, Multiple sclerosis: fat-oil relationship, nutrition 1991, Sep-Oct; 7(5):368-375.

Swank (1961) "Biochemical basis of MS" Springfield IL, Charles Thomas pub.

Pritikin references:

Armstrong (1970) *"Regression of coronary atheromatosis in rhesus monkeys" circ res 27:59.*

Kuo (1955) **"Angina pectoris induced by fat ingestion** in patients with coronary artery disease" JAMA 158: 1008-13.

Friedman (1965) **"Effect of unsaturated fats upon lipemia & conjunctival circulation**" JAMA 193: 882-86.

Winitz (1970) "Studies in metaboloic nutrition employing **chemically defined diets**" Amer J clin nutr 23: 525-45

McKean (1970) "Grow of phenylketonuric children on **chemically defined diets**" Lancet I:148

Whyte (1958) "Body fat and BP of natives of **New Guinea**" Austr ann med, 7:36-45

Leaf (1971) "Hard labor, low chol, linked to longevity" Med tribune, June

Page (1970) **"Prediction of coronary ht dz based on age, total chol, TG"** Circ. 42: 625-45

Blankenhorn (1978) "Rate of atherosclerosis change during Tx of hyperlipoproteinemia" circ 57:355-61.

Astrup (1973) "CO, smoking, & CV dz" circ 48: 1167-68. Lowering blood oxygen only 15-20% caused increased endothelial permeability & subintimal edema.

Sweeney (1927) "Dietary factors that influence dextrose tolerance test" Arch int med, 40: 818-30.

Goldblatt (1953) **"Induced malignancy in rat subjected to anaerobiosis"** j exp med 97:525-52.

Warburg "Prime cause and prevention of cancer" editor Dean Burk, **35% reduction of O2 was able to induce cancer**.

Pritikin, Nathan "Pritikin Program of diet & exercise" book, copyright 1979 [has great summary of lipotoxemia theory]. & "Review of Medical Literature" copyright 1988 [legacy book summarizing his work], (available at Dr McDougall dot com).

Brasky, Theodore (2013) "Plasma phospholipid fatty acids and prostate cancer risk in the SELECT TRIAL." Nat'l cancer institute. Aug 7; 105 (15): 1132-41.

Griffini et al. (1998) "Dietary omega 3 promote colon cancer metastases in rat liver." cancer res, Aug 1: 58 (15): 3312-19

Chapter 21. **<u>About the author</u>**

Peter Rogers MD is the Nostredamus of nutrition, the Spartan Vegan, the Bad Boy of veganism, the Medical Monk, the Messiah of Metabolism, Plant Man Prometheus, the Vegan Prophet, Modern Diogenes, Dutch Uncle, Medical Heretic, and so on.

"Dr Rogers has the most comprehensive, and accurate understanding of pathophysiology [disease causation] of anyone in the world" – Gregory Sloop MD, best atherosclerosis researcher in the world.

Dr Rogers makes the **you tube channel "Peter Rogers MD,"** and also posts some videos at Rumble, Bit Chute, Linked In & Facebook. He will go to these places and Odysee if he gets booted off YT.

To contact Dr Rogers, you can send an email to **rogersmd@protonmail.com.**

Dr Rogers is the author of about 20 books, including **"the Medical Reformation: poor man's guide to health, nutrition & toxicology,"** as well as many other books including **"Holy Grail of Wisdom Quotes," "Best Christian Art," "How to raise IQ & become a genius," "Straight A at Stanford and on to Harvard"** and others.

Peter Rogers MD graduated first in his medical school class, and had 99% board scores in medical school & residency. He did a surgical internship, and then obtained board certifications in diagnostic radiology, interventional radiology (imaging guided surgery), and neuroradiology.

Dr Rogers got fat in his mid 30's and Dr McDougall's advice on the starch diet helped him to lose all the weight from 220 lbs, down to 154 lbs. He was featured on the Dr McDougall.com website as a Star McDougaller.

Dr Rogers is the pioneer of the ischemic spinal degeneration theory (the best theory of spinal degeneration), as being a diffuse process.

Roger's theory shows that spinal degeneration includes more than DDD (degenerative disc disease), but also interbody fusion, DISH (diffuse idiopathic skeletal hyperostosis), OPLL (ossification of posterior longitudinal ligament), OLF (ossification of ligamentum flavum), and Baastrup's disease (posterior spinous process fusion), and how this relates to weak ligaments from collagen damage by F- and to GP, and by a lack of vitamin C.

He is the discoverer of the neuro-vascular uncoupling (NVU) theory of brain degeneration; also called the supply and demand theory of dementia. This is the best theory of dementia.

He figured out the role of mitochondrial inhibitors in the causation of dementia, and cancer.

219

He figured out how the nutrition guidelines for TBI (traumatic brain injury) and stroke should be rewritten to include more dietary fiber to protect both the gut barrier and the blood brain barrier.

He is also the author of books about art, literature, and study skills.

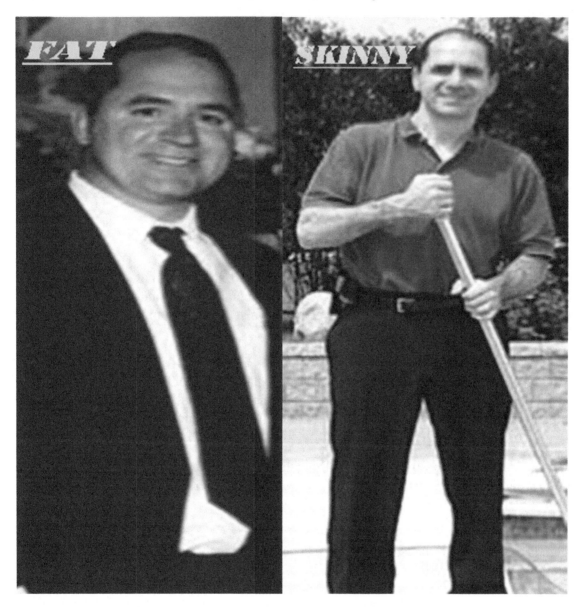

Fig 21-1: Dr Rogers got fat in his 30's and struggled with the weight for 3 years, before learning about the McDougall diet. He then lost all the weight, from 220 lbs, down to 154 lbs, and became a "star McDougaller," featured on Dr McDougall's website, Dr McDougall dot com.

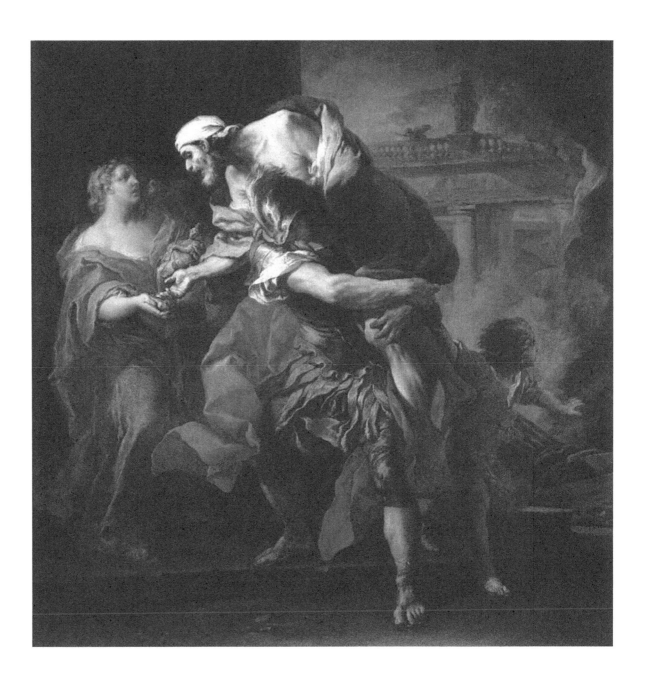

Fig 21-2: **Aeneas carrying his father Anchises out of burning Troy** by Carl van Loo, 1729, public domain.

"The best a man can do is to learn about the good things in civilization and try to transmit this to the next generation.

If a man is fortunate he will before he dies, gather up as much as he can of his civilized heritage and transmit it to his children.

And to his final breath he will be grateful for this inexhaustible legacy, knowing that it is our nourishing mother and our lasting life." - Will Durant.

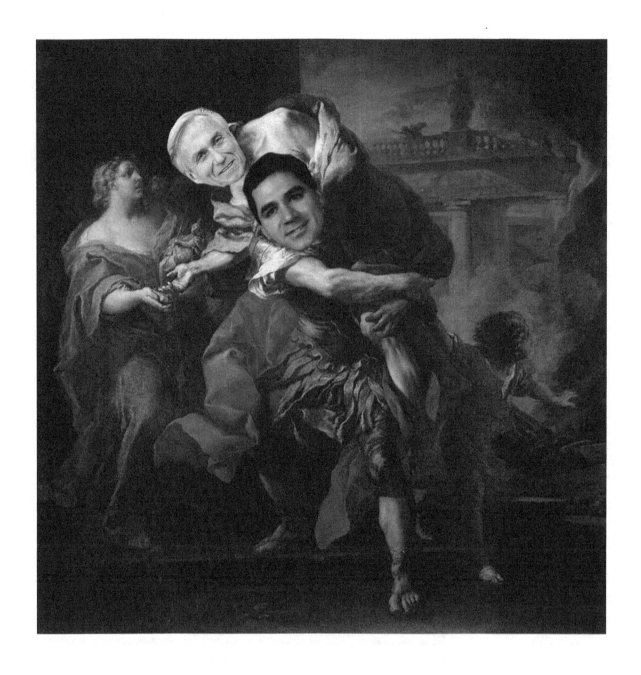

Fig 21-3: Aeneas carrying his father Anchises out of burning Troy by Carl van Loo, 1729, public domain. **Dr Rogers carrying his intellectual father, Dr McDougall, out of modern chaos.**

Dr McDougall: Put me down! You little upstart!

Dr Rogers: I'm just carrying your legacy.

Dr McDougall: I can carry it myself! I'm the fighting Irish!

Dr Rogers: I know you can, but I wanted to try to help.

222

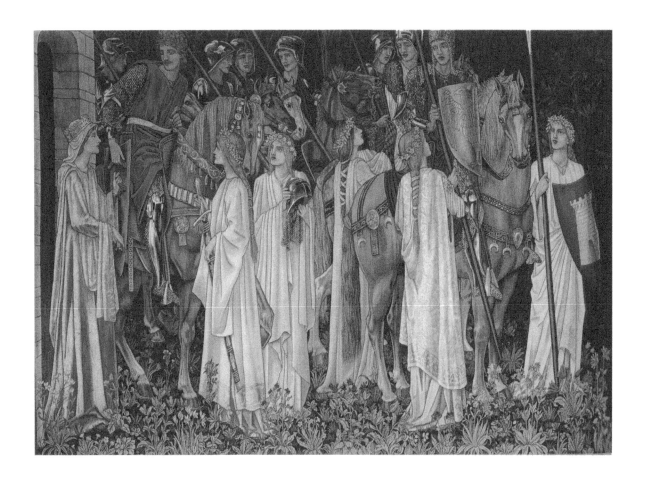

Fig 21-4: **Departure of the Knights** by Edward Burne Jones, 1870, public domain. The students of Dr McDougall must rise to the challenge; to teach the truth of nutrition; to maintain the legacy of Dr McDougall.

Index

Abdominal pressure syndrome

academic orgasm 53

ACLM 41

acid load on kidneys 178

aging 189

alkaline 180

aluminum 174-175

alzheimer disesae 174

angioplasty see chapter on heart disease

anspaugh, Jean Renfro author of fat like us 82

antacids 191

arsenic 80-81

asian populations 98

asthma 151

atherosclerosis see chapter on heart disease

atrial fibrillation 170

autism 158

autoimmune disease see chapter on autoimmune disease

B

babies & baby feeding 183-184

B12 94

Bantu women and lack of osteoporosis 62

benzoate 185

blindness 184, 194

bone mineral density see chapter on osteoporosis

breath bad 106

breast cancer 24, 141

breast milk humans 183

bridging molecules 90

Burkitt, Dennis 4, 68-72

butyrate 107

C

CABG 162

ceres 187

caloric density 118

cancer 141

cardiology 45

carnivore diet 162, 189

calcium 3,

calcium channel blocker 130

campbell 30, 94

cataracts 156, 184

cholesterol 117 (hdl), 125, 164

cme 27

coffee 192

comparitive anatomy 55

connor, Wm 58

copper see chapter on dementia

crohns 108

cystitis, interstitial 152

D

dairy 124, 156, 182

dante 28-29, 83

dementia see chapter on dementia

denmark 190

Deodorants

diabetes 103, 105, 134

diet comparison chart ii, 4-11, 4-12

disclaimer 5

doctor diet 26

don quixote (DQ)32-33-34-36-37

donnison paper 61

drug companies 23

dyes in food 185

E

Epidemiology 55

eskimos 103, 169, 181

esselstyn 66, 94

estrogen therapy 147

exams physical annual 192

exercise 190

F

Fat high fat meal

fat is bad 94

fats "good" 109

fat lowers po2 2, causes blood sludge 2,

fat plant foods 3

Feingold diet 185

fractures see chapter on osteoporosis

finland 4-9

fish oil 103

fluorosis 183

friedman 92

fruits 3, 121,

G

Gallstones 109

gladiators 55

glycemic index 195

Gotzsche 143

gout 151

grains 187

Gruntzig 38

gum disease 175

gut wall 107

H

heart disease – see chapter on heart disease

History 55

hrt 182

hyperparathyroidism 152

Hypertension 126

I

ibd 108

ibs 108

ilgf 181

immune system 142

Impotence

infants and infant feeding 183-184

Iron 172

Insurance companies 23

Ivy college image 57

J

Japan

jurek 58

K

Kempner 48, 73-80, 82-83, 122-123, 131

Kempner diet 4

Kenya 4-5, 4-6

227

kidney -see chapter on kidneys and osteoporosis, 178

kuo 92

L

LDL cholesterol see cholesterol

leaky gut 107, 159

liver fatty 109

lipemia 168-169

longevity 55

lose weight 116

low carb diet 162, 189

Lundberg 197

lungs 190

lung cancer screening 190

lymphoma 147-148

M

mammography see chapter on cancer

Mcdougall, Christopher, author of born to run 4-4

Mcdougall diet 53, 119, 193

methionine 64

migration studies 55

Mitochondria inhibitors

moderation 112

Mood 175, 190

Moore, Richard 132

Multiple sclerosis see swank

mummy 56

muscle 103

N

Nelson, Jeff foreword, 66

Newsletter archive 8

Nuts 170

O

Oils 101-102, 114-116, 170

Okinawa 62, 98

omega 3 2, 103, 114, 115-116, 125, 136, 170, 173

osteoarthritis 160

osteonecrosis 195

osteopenia see chapter on osteoporosis

Osteoporosis see chapter on osteoporosis and kidneys

oxalates 181

P

Paintings & drawings: God speed by Leeighton fron cover and 2-1,Dr Mcdougall fights big meat I, comparison chart of diets ii, starch is best food iii, Mcdougall archives of newsletters 1-1, starch solution cover 1-2, digestive tune up cover 1-3, healthiest diet on the planet 1-4, Mcdougall's medicine book cover 1-5, Mcdougall program for heart cover 1-6, Mcdougall program for weight loss 1-7, Mcdougall book for women 1-8, the dedication by Leighton 2-2, Accolade by Leighton 2-3, reception at versailles by Gerome 2-4, Sir Galahad by Hughes 2-5, Gates of hell by blake 2-6, dante with divine comedy by Michelino 2-7, Maid milking cow by Borch 2-8, DQ in library 2-9, DQ speech 2-10, Priest and barber in DQ library by Balaca 2-11, time of peril by leighton 2-12, DQ and SP on the trails by Detti 2-13, DQ fights windmill 2-14, fighting knights by Delacroix 2-15, Faded laurels by Leighton 2-16, the bard martin 2-17, star mcdougallers 3-1, starch solution 3-2, digestiv etuneup 3-3, starch is low caloric density 4-1, tarahumara map 4-2, pima 4-3, bordiet comparison chart 4-11, n to run by CM 4-4), Keny map 4-5, HTN Donnison paper 4-6, Bantu women 4-7, Okinawa 4-8, Finland 4-9, diet comparison descriptions 4-12, abdominal pressure syndrome 5-1, burkitt biography 5-2, kempner weigh in 5-3, kempner harem 5-4, kempner eye improvements 5-4, Kempner chest xray improvements 5-5, kempner table of contents 5-6, kempner biography 5-7, fat like us by anspaugh 5-8, swank book on ms 5-9, swank paper on md 34 yr followup 5-10, swank paper on sat fat 5-11, mcdougall blood sludge video 5-12, blood sludge drawing 5-13, zeta potential 5-14, bridging molecutes 5-15 , Peter Kuo paper graph 5-16, pritikn book toc 5-17, starch solution cover 6-1, starch drawing 6-2, digestive tuneup 7-1, Gulliver by Vibert 7-2, leaky gut 7-3, battle of bulge movie cover 8-1, caloric density drawing 8-2, cancer doubling time 11-1, leaky gut 12-1, my fair lady 19-1, King Arthur 19-2, round table of dr mcdougall (and king arthur) 19-3, death of king arthur by Archer 19-4, death of king arrthur by scott 19-5, peter rogers star mcdougaller 21-1, aeneas carries anchises 21-2, rogers carries mcdougall 21-3, departure of the knights (students) 21-4

paleo diet 162, 189

paleontology 56, 120-121, 191

Papua New Guinea

Parkinson disease 152, 172

pima 57

polyps 108

polychondritis 159

potassium 132

potatos 120, see chapter on potatos 199

pregnancy 184

Prostate see chapter on cancer

PSA see chapter on cancer

pral 178

pritikin 58, 93-96, 203

protein 3

Psoriasis 153

pump head 168

Q

Quotes dk simonton 16, swift 16, schopenhauer 16, holmes 17, fleming 17, cajal 17, 2nd timothy 19, carnap 24, plato 27, orwell 27, augustine 37, dostoevsky 37, emerson 41-2, jung 93, wilde 113,

R

RBC size

rheumatoid arthritis see chapter on autoimmune disease

Rice 80-81

risk absolute vs relative 195

Rogers, Peter quotes 60

rosenman 92

runners 56

S

SAD diet = standard american diet

salmon 64

sarcopenia 185

sb 380 41

scfa 107

schizophrenia 153, 158

set point 123

sleep apnea 190

sludge blood 88-89-92, 116

sodium 84, 129

soy 102, 181

standard of care 20

star macougallers 49

Starch is the solution 1, 53

Starch drawing 6, 54, 100

statins see chapter on heart disease, 170, 185

stents 23, see chapter on heart disease

sulfur 108

Sunshine

Swank 85-88

sweeteners artificial 126

T

Tarahumara 57

testosterone therapy 147

thyroid 157

triglycerides 117

U

ulcerative colitis 108, 153

Uric acid

V

Vitamin B12

vitamin d 191

W

website of dr mcdougall 8

weight how to lose 117

widowmaker 167

wikipedia 38

X

Y

Yanomamo

Z

Zeta potential 90

Notes:

Notes:

Notes:

Notes:

Made in the USA
Las Vegas, NV
25 August 2024